A Tale of Healthcare Fraud and Abuse
A Nursing Home Administrator Blows the Whistle

By

Joseph Wellington, Ph.D.

Day 30 (Resignation)

"Well, if you won't, then we'll find someone who will. It's your choice," the regional director of operations said. He was a short man with large brimmed black glasses. He wore a faded, and somewhat yellowing, white button up shirt with wrinkled black pants. Underneath his black yarmulke was an unwashed head of hair and beneath that was a body that hadn't showered in days.

Samuel, or Shmuey as everyone called him, was the nephew of the nursing home's owner. He had very little education, dressed and spoke unprofessionally, and perhaps mostly importantly, was untouchable.

On that fateful day, I was sitting across the desk looking at him in disbelief. Five minutes prior to his empty threat was a discussion over financial statements that were misleading, at best. "You are the licensed provider and you are required to sign these financials," he said without any understanding of his own statement.

"Shmuey, with all do respect, I cannot sign these financials. They are inaccurate. In fact, they read that this building is highly profitable when, in fact, this facility is hemorrhaging cash. If signing these documents is so important, why don't you sign these documents? I have only been here for a month anyway and these statements are two months old," I said.

I reached for the bottom of my necktie and rolled it up and down the bottom half of my stomach while bouncing my right leg. My heartbeat sped up and the office somehow became a much warmer place, evidenced by the sweat accumulating under my arms.

"Dr. Wellington, Joseph is going to be pissed about this. You are fucking with the wrong owner here. You know damn well that we cannot sign this document and you are refusing to do your job. How the fuck am I supposed to go back to Joseph's office and tell him that you refused to sign, huh?" As if it weren't bad enough that he was difficult to look at before, he was now red with veins bulging from his neck. Hey may not have wanted to physically hit me but to the onlooker, it would have appeared that way.

Joseph was a very well known nursing home owner. He had been known for many things including screaming at administrators, throwing coffee mugs across the room, and demanding full submission to his will. Shmuey feared Joseph more than he feared god. Many people did.

I stood up from the wheeled leather chair and leaned over the desk while placing my hands for support. This was my 'position of power'. We looked directly into each other's eyes for what seemed to be hours. The smell of his body odor set the tone for better urgency to halt. Then, I turned away and pushed the speakerphone button on the black telephone.

"How may I help you Dr. Wellington," came the disembodied voice from the telephone speaker. "Jane, please alert Tom in maintenance that I shall require a box for my belongings."

"What? Is this a joke," Jane said. Jane and I became closely working colleagues over the month I was employed. Like all good assistants, she even knew my spouse's birthday within the first week. She was truly one of the best.

"I'm afraid it is not a joke. Additionally, I will need you to alert the human resources department that I need a copy of the payroll to date for my records."

"Right away sir."

I glanced over at Shmuey, "Then I guess you will have to do what you have to do." And, with that statement, I walked over to the bookshelf and removed personal pictures and three books on regulatory compliance. I created a small pile on my desk. "You're a real asshole, you know that," he said.

Then, I looked at him without hesitation, "This is excellent news for me. I am no longer bound by the facility's confidentiality clause. Please pass along a message to your beloved Joseph. There is a storm coming. Every secret I am aware of will become knowledge of regulators within the next forty-eight hours."

Shmuey grabbed and stroked his very short brown beard. He moved his yarmulke from side to side on his head. Then, he reached for the telephone on my desk. I swiftly pulled the cord out of the telephone. "This is still my office and until I leave, my rules will apply in here. You will need to ask to use the telephone and, at the moment, I'm not giving permission. I'll be gone within the next ten minutes. Then, feel free to do whatever it is that you want to do in here." Shmuey sat back in the chair. He was not willing to challenge me any further.

I sat down in my leather chair and turned to the computer. I highlighted all emails and hit the delete button. The computer took a short amount of time to process such a large amount of deletions while the hourglass on the screen turned repeatedly. Watching this hourglass turn was somehow soothing. My heartbeat returned to normal and I no longer had racing thoughts and angry emotions. Then, I deleted the trash folder. This deletion went much faster and then I clicked 'shut down' on the screen. The screen went black and my image was visible in the reflection.

Tom knocked at the door and I waved at him through the glass to enter. He walked in with a storage file box that had been emptied. "Dr. Wellington, this sucks. We were really starting to like you." He turned and looked at Shmuey with squinted eyes and a smug facial expression. "What can I do to help you get packed sir?" Tom was over six foot tall with graying blonde hair. He was thin and his face weathered from all the years wearing down his body in this line of work. But, Tom's face was one of sincere compassion and concern. He was the paternal type to everyone.

He set the box down on the office conference table and looked around the room to see what belongings were mine. "Everything I own is on this desk. If you wouldn't mind helping me with these, that would be great. I'm waiting on the payroll report from human resources before I officially leave the facility. The flowers on the conference table are also mine and I'll grab those last."

Shmuey sat quietly in the chair he never moved from the entire time. He stared at his iPhone while typing and reading. Although he may have been communicating the current situation to the corporate office, it appeared to me that this was a comfort tool for him. His anger had turned to nervousness. He had a good reason to be nervous.

I handed my car key to Tom and asked him to take the box of items and the flowers to my car. He collected the belongings and proceeded out of the office taking long strides. As he exited, Jane entered in her usual color coordinated outfit of reds with matching high heels. Her reading glasses are the only item that gives away her age being over forty. "Dr. Wellington, is there anything I can do for you before you leave? I'm going to really miss you." She walked over to me and hugged me tightly. "You take good care of yourself, okay?" I hugged her back. As she walked out of the office, she turned around and said, "I forgot to mention your new tie is amazing." I looked at my tie and realized the design was SpongeBob SquarePants, picked out by my children. I laughed and then she laughed. Then, I sat down and remained quiet.

"Is there a reason you are still here, Joseph," came from a smugly toned voice across the desk. He was no longer stroking his beard and playing with his yarmulke. His arms were folded across his chest and his iPhone sat in front of him on my now nearly empty desk.

"Yes."

There was a long pause. He looked at me and I looked back over at him.

"What the hell do you want now? You want me to give you a round of fucking applause as you exit the facility?"

"No. I am waiting for the mid-payroll period report for my records. I want to make sure that when someone complains that you 'trimmed' their paychecks I have the reports to prove they are right."

"You are not entitled to those fucking reports and you know it. You are quitting."

"I'm not leaving here without those reports. And, while we are on the subject of things that we are and are not entitled to, you should know that I am no longer obligated to keep your personal secrets, either. You know, ones like you having an affair with the director of nursing at this facility. Or, the falsification of records to cover up Mr. Jones' death after the dialysis clamp failed because it was never applied correctly. This is just the beginning."

"You are really fucking pissing me off, man. Luckily for you, I just got a text message from Joseph asking me to get you to sign a confidentiality agreement in return for a $10,000 severance payment."

"This isn't about your money. You just don't get it do you? This was about me being here less than a month with a goal of trying to get this company to go on the straight and narrow to get things done correctly. But, then you badgered me to illegally sign a document and threatened me. Even if I were so inclined to take this confidentiality 'bribe', it would certainly be worth a lot more than $10,000. Tell him, I'm absolutely not interested."

Shmuey snatched his iPhone from the desk and put his face very close to the screen while he pounded the glass. His angry typing made me wonder if his fingers were hurting. The room once again went silent when he put his iPhone down. Then, the sound of buzzing came from the desk. He picked up his iPhone and read the message out loud to me, "Then you can tell Dr. Fuckface that if he blabs about our internal workings we'll see him in court. He can take the fucking money or we'll destroy him."

"Ha! That is all you guys have? As soon as I get my report, I'll be out of your hair for the rest of the day. I'm not threatening you. You're being told that I'm filing the complaints so that you don't terminate someone that you 'assume' is filing them to protect yourselves. This way, you know where they are coming from."

He started pounded hard on the iPhone again when I heard a meek knock on the glass window in the door. I looked up and waved at Mary to enter. She carried a plain manila file folder with the documents inside of them. The label on the folder indicated that it was the mid-payroll period report for pay period ending xx-xx-xxxx. She was scrupulously organized. "Dr. Wellington, here are the reports you have requested. I was told over the phone that you are leaving us, effective today. Have you put this in writing?"

"I have not put this in writing. For professional reasons, I cannot tell you why I will not put this in writing but I can only tell you that no written notice will be provided today. But, it has been a real pleasure to have worked with such an organized professional like you."

Mary came to the other side of the desk and put her arms around me like a mother would to her son while I remained seated. She smelled of rose perfume and wore turquoise jewelry. Her hug was firm and comforting. "We're going to miss you around here." Then, she turned around and, without acknowledging that Shmuey was even in the room, marched out of the office and pulled the door shut behind her.

I stood up and leaned over the desk to plug the phone cord back into the phone. "You may now use my telephone if you are so inclined. Please consider this my resignation. You will not get it in writing because I am leaving because of a request to compromise my integrity and break the law. As angry as I am with you, I hope that you can find someone that will meet the cultural norms you are looking for in this facility."

Shmuey replied in the most unprofessional manner, one in which I had grown accustomed to from him, by simply saying, "Oh fuck off." He stood up and turned my direction. His shirt was even more wrinkled from his arms being crossed.

I grabbed my blazer and held it over one arm while carrying the file folder. I walked out of the office and closed the door behind me. A fax machine loudly printed a document. And, the heat of the printing was overpowering. I said 'goodbye' to many of the office workers and exited the facility for the last time.

Pre-Employment

"Hello. This is Joseph," I said answering the Blackberry that was always attached to my hip.

"Hi Joseph. My name is Sarah and I am the corporate human resources director for JAR Management. I'm terribly sorry to call you the day before Christmas but Joseph Rackman asked me to give you a call and……"

I interrupted her, "Joseph who? What is this in regards to?"

"Mr. Rackman would like to offer you the position of nursing home administrator for a property near your home. I believe you met him during an interview six months ago. Are you currently employed?"

"Okay, I'm sorry for the confusion. I did meet Joseph a while back and no I'm not currently working. I decided to take a year off and work on postdoctoral studies. What facility are you calling about?"

"That is where it gets a little tricky. The facility is called xxxxxxxx Care Center and it is exactly two miles from your home. It is one of our most challenging facilities, though. We currently have three weeks until the facility is decertified. When the state was in last week, they mentioned that you would be a perfect fit for this position."

I took a deep breath and sighed audibly. The state department of health never recommends a specific administrator for any facility because of the conflict of interest. This was a telephone call of desperation. Immediately, the thought of salary crossed my mind since it was not mentioned, as of yet.

"Wow. That is shocking and certainly flattering. I wonder which surveyors recommended me? I have known most of them for many years now. Let's talk about timeframe and salary here. I'm a little concerned about the very short deadline to clear this facility from noncompliance and payment of my salary if the facility gets decertified."

There was a long pause on the other end of this telephone call. It was clear she knew that I was not a 'newbie' at this sort of negotiation. Then, she responded in a very calculated manner, "Mr. Rackman is prepared to offer you a salary of $65,000 per year plus a $25,000 bonus for clearing the facility of the deficiencies. And, of course....."

I interrupted with laughter. She had to be joking about the salary. "You have got to be joking. I made that salary 15 years ago and you are willing to offer that to me today. I'm sorry I don't think I'm the right candidate for this job. You are obviously looking for someone fresh out of an associate's degree program with absolutely no experience whatsoever. Thank you for thinking of me, though."

"Absolutely not. Mr. Rackman has demanded that I secure you for this facility, specifically. These surveyors want you. This team needs you. What numbers can we negotiate to get this to work?" The desperation showed through the phone. Her breathing was heavy as if she were overweight at the beginning of this call and now it was heavily labored. She was nervous.

"I will not accept this position without an agreement as an independent contract with an up front retainer of $30,000 until the facility clears. Once the facility clears the deficiencies, if I agree to stay on board, I will be looking at a salary of $125,000 per year with an executive compensation package to be negotiated at that time."

"Done."

"Please forward that, in writing, to my email address and we have a deal. Of course, I'll need to have the retainer check within 48 hours, as well. You may make the check out to Joseph Wellington, Ph.D."

"The email will go out later today and I'll have a check overnighted to your home. Please respond with your correct mailing address once you get the email, though."

"Let's talk specifics about this home and what it needs. Are you the person I need to speak with or should I be talking to the regional director of operations here?"

There was a long pause and I was certain that she had terminated the telephone call. Over the years, I had become accustomed to human resources professionals attempting to describe operational issues. It never worked out. She clearly called me with the intention of getting a 'yes' answer without any negotiation. I worried that she was emotionally exhausted by this very short conversation, thus far.

But, then, I could hear talking in the background. The voices all seemed oddly loud. "Who wants to field this one," came a voice that clearly was on the line. Gasp! I was on a conference call.

So, in a very polite manner I said, "Is this a conference call? If this was a conference call, I should have been made aware of that when the call first opened up. Let me get a pen and paper so that I can write down the names of everyone here. Okay, now if everyone can please tell me their names and positions so that I know who I am addressing that would be great."

The call went silent again. There were absolutely no voices this time. I looked down and wrote, '*On the Line*' and then underlined it. The next line, I carefully wrote, '*Sarah from JAR Management*'. On the far right corner of the page, I wrote, '*xxxxxxx Care Center*' and the date. Then, I clicked the pen closed and put it down.

"Dr. Wellington, I'm sorry to keep you waiting. There are five of us on this call. We should have told you that when the call started and we do apologize for this."

"Please feel free to call me Joseph. May I ask who I am speaking with?"

"My name is Frank Frankl and I am the general counsel for JAR Management."

I picked up the pen quickly and wrote, '*Frank Frankl, General Counsel*'. Then, I asked, "Would everyone else please identify themselves now? I'm writing this down. If we're all going to work together, it shouldn't be a problem anyway."

"Joseph, it's Frank again. The following people are on the line. There is Sarah Dustfy, our human resources director, Sarah Mendelbaum, our human resources assistant, Shmuey Rackman, our regional director of operations for that region, Julie Storey, our reimbursement specialist for that region, and Latisha Howard, the regional corporate nurse for the property we are talking about."

I grabbed my pen and started jotting down all of the names phonetically. I was unsure of how to spell 'Shmuey', 'Mendelbaum', and 'Dustfy' but that was simply not important at this time. A lot of voices came all at once, "We're all here."

"Aren't any of you lunkheads listening on this call? I was merely identifying all of you," Frank said. His voice was tense and loud. The word 'lunkheads' was one I had not heard in a very long time and it was somehow comforting to hear that used towards others instead of myself. "We're sorry Frank. Let's get started."

The phone call got crowded out with voices. Everyone was talking at once and I was unable to make out any sense out of the garbled sounds. "Hello, I can't understand anything on this call with everyone talking at once. I tell you what, may I ask specific questions of specific people so that we can make this more orderly."

"Of course, Dr. Wellington," came a very sweet and timid female voice, "Please proceed."

"First and foremost, I will need someone to scan and send me copies of the statement of deficiencies. I would like that sent to me this evening with the signed contract via email. Who will take care of this?"

The call fell silent again. "Okay, folks. Don't everyone speak up at once. I'd be lying if I said I wasn't feeling a little bit of pressure at the moment with this timeline. I'm going to need a lot more cooperation so that we can move quickly here."

A very gruff sounding voice with a heavy accent came on the line, "Joseph, I'll get those items over to you shortly. Sarah, do you have Joseph's email address?" The voice never identified himself. So, I said, "May I ask who I'm speaking with?"

"It's Shmuey. Look, don't feel so much pressure. Now that you are here, we know we'll clear. We have a lot of faith in you."

"Thanks. Now, let's talk briefly about what the major issues are here."

"Joseph, can we do that tomorrow. I'd like to meet with you at the facility. Can you be there?"

"I will be at the facility at 8am," I said. Shmuey, however, quickly responded with, "I can't get there that early. The earliest I can be there will be 11."

"Okay, I'll be there at 11. Is there anything else we need to cover on this call?"

"No. I think that's it for now," Frank said.

"Very good. I'll look forward to seeing the signed contract in my email box this evening, along with the statement of deficiencies. Then I'll be there tomorrow at 11am."

"Thank you for helping us Dr. Wellington," came a very meek voice again. But, I never did ask who this was.

I pulled my Blackberry from my ear and hit the 'End Call' button with my index finger. The red notification light started blinking right away. So, I typed in the password and opened the email box. There, in front of me, was an email marked 'Urgent' from Sarah Dustfy with an attachment laying out the terms of our agreement. It was a scanned copy of the agreement that had been signed by Joseph Rackman and Frank Frankl. Joseph Rackman's signature was easy to read but Frank Frankl's signature was only identifiable by his typed name underneath the signature line.

The message was then marked 'unread' so that I could print this out from the computer later and the Blackberry placed back in my hip holster.

That evening, I sat down in my home office and wrote in my journal: '*JAR Management team called today and asked for my help. They started out with a lie that the public health officials requested my services, specifically. Then they tried to lowball my salary. Why in the world did I agree to start working with them after they threw a lot of money at me? I'm starting to work on contract with JAR Management tomorrow in a very challenging facility that requires a full turnaround. The corporate team is unresponsive, irresponsible, and indifferent to this facility or its needs – this is the problem, not the facility. I'm worried. The money, however, is very good. If I don't like it, I'll refund the unused part of the retainer and leave. What an odd team. This is going to be a real rollercoaster ride.*'

Day 1

The next day, Christmas Day to be precise, I arrived at the facility at 11am. The parking lot was nearly empty and the front lobby was all the same. The lobby was nothing impressive, either. It had a few chairs, a flat blue carpet, and a brass lamp. There was also a plastic runner.

While the receptionist desk remained empty, I decided to push the small desk bell for help. Then I waited. After a few moments, I pushed the bell again. This time, the front door to the facility slid open and in walked a man wearing a long black wool business coat and a black fedora. "Are you Joseph," he said in a gruff voice. I immediately recognized him as Shmuey from this sound.

"I am Joseph, Shmuey. It is a pleasure to meet you in person."

"Follow me. I'll take you to your new office and fill you in on a few details of the facility. Will you need a tour of the property before you take the reigns today?"

I chuckled in the firm belief that this was a joke. "Why is that funny," he said in a very serious tone. "I thought you were making a joke. Yes, I will need a full tour of the property along with the life safety code portions and a copy of the disaster plan before I get started."

We walked around the receptionist's desk and into an office with a glass window built into the door. The heat was not working in this office and I left my coat on. Shmuey, being a much larger man, removed his coat immediately and tossed it over one of the conference chairs. "I didn't get the statement of deficiencies via email last night and I will need that." His facial expressions were smug and angry. I contemplated leaving at that very minute.

"I want to talk to you about that but after we finish the tour."

"Okay."

The office was disorganized with papers on the floor. The desk had a dusty computer that resembled everything else. Papers lined the desks in piles and the floor had not been vacuumed in some time. The administrator's desk chair was an institutional dining room chair. "You can leave your coat in here. We don't have any thefts here so there is nothing to worry about," he said calmly.

"Even it were not cold in here, I wouldn't remove my coat and place it on a chair. When is the last time this office has seen a housekeeper? Has anyone used this office recently? And, more importantly, why would anyone want to stay when the welcome to this facility is brought with this horrid example?"

After looking at me momentarily and smiling he responded, "You got me there. We haven't had any housekeeping services for any of the offices. We cut the housekeeping staff to save money and now we can barely get the resident care areas cleaned. All staff are responsible to clean their own offices."

"And, how is that working out?"

"You are witness to how that is working out."

"Okay, well let's get the party started. Just let me grab a pen." I followed him out of the door and into the nursing home to begin the tour. The first floor was beautiful with shiny new wallpaper, newly installed premium wooden doors, soft lighting, new state of the art equipment and designer furniture, and residents that moved about the facility without the use of a wheelchair. The first floor also contained an in-house dialysis program and large therapy gymnasium with state of the art equipment.

Each office window I peered through was dirty and the sight behind them was not much different. The garbage cans overflowed, the desks were disorganized, and the floors were dirty. And, while offices are usually locked to protect patient health information privacy, none of the offices were locked.

The second floor was quite different. The bottom half of the walls were painted with a light brown paint while the top half were painted with a dark green. The walls were scuffed from wheelchairs and other paraphernalia. The hallways were dark and dreary with lights the flickered. The ceiling tiles were yellow in many spots, and had water stains in many areas, and the tracking to this ceiling was rusted. There were holes in many of these tiles. Exit signs flickered at the end of each hallway.

While the first floor elevator entrance was lined with beautiful mahogany, the second floor elevator entrance was painted and scuffed with pen marks and dirt. The dining room adjacent to the elevator had white floor tile that had yellowed and lot its ability to retain any sort of shine.

The residents on this floor were missing socks and shoes, wore dirty clothing and some only wore a hospital gown, many drooled while having difficulty holding their heads up from their wheelchairs. Unlike the first floor, this floor had a strong odor of urine and feces. The dining rooms had strong body odors.

The second floor bedrooms had furniture that was old and dilapidated. The in-room heaters were not secured to the walls in many rooms as cracks were visible to the outside of the facility. The walls had lots of patching, very little paint that had been faded, and lots of holes.

And, to make matters worse, while walking through resident rooms, we noticed that there was only one staff member for the entire floor of 140 residents. She was a nurse that refused to do any 'hands on resident care' – or as we termed it changing residents when they are soiled, dressing them, and assisting them with bathing.

Shmuey walked through the halls and didn't speak to anyone. He matter-of-factly pointed to elevator rooms, mechanical rooms, dialysis rooms, therapy rooms, and resident rooms. Staff members that were present on the first floor didn't speak to him. The one staff member on the second floor didn't speak to him. I wondered, internally, if the staff members even knew who he was and, if so, why they were not speaking to him. It was all so confusing.

We returned to the administrator's office and sat down at the round conference table. Shmuey pulled out a file with the statement of deficiencies inside. Then, he lowered his voice, "There is no way we will clear all of these tags. It is just not going to fucking happen. I don't know why they think you are going to be a fucking miracle worker but you ain't. So, on Monday, if the state arrives you are going to give me a call and I'm going to bring cash. We're going to pull the lead surveyor into the office and tell them that we're willing to pay whatever it takes."

"Whoa! Are you saying that you are going to bribe the surveyor? I want no part of that."

"Don't be so naïve. We do this all of the time and we can't afford to take a gamble on you."

"So, why in the world am I even here?"

"We need an administrator in the building that the surveyors are familiar with. If they take the cash, they will feel comfortable knowing that you can fix the building later without their bosses become suspicious."

"I see. So, I'm being used as the offering?" He merely nodded his head. "Okay, I'll accept that but I will not until the check clears for the retainer."

"Why are you so fucking concerned about a retainer check? Don't you have enough money and can't you feel for our situation here? We're struggling with all of the fines being levied against us."

"And, that, Shmuey is exactly why I am concerned about the retainer check. I have had this situation happen before where I don't get paid. No sir. This will not happen this time around. I'll take a look at the statement of deficiencies and I need a set of keys for the facility." He pulled out an extra set of keys and a sheet of paper. "Please sign this form acknowledging that you received these keys." I reviewed and signed.

I looked over at the clock, 2:45pm. "Wow, the time flew by fast. Let's say we call it a day. I need to review all of these documents and start formulating a plan. Do you have the telephone number for the human resources director so that I can have access to staffing patterns here? I noticed that there are very few staff members for such a large number of residents."

He walked over to the hutch of the administrator's desk and pulled out a binder. The binder contained the telephone numbers of all staff with their titles. "I won't call her today because of Christmas but I will give her a call tomorrow. I also intend to be here tomorrow." Shmuey dressed himself with his coat and hat and proceeded out of the administrator's office. He never bid me adieu or any other cliché goodbye. He merely walked out of the door.

I stayed behind to review the statement of deficiencies. The deficiencies were severe: facility acquired wounds, administering the wrong medications that resulted in resident injury, administering the wrong amounts of insulin, unmanaged falls, not notifying the physician when the resident had changes in condition, and others. The facility's lack of leadership from the corporate office created an absolute mess.

One deficiency that struck me as concerning, and easily fixed, was the administration of an incorrect amount of insulin. I decided to conduct a small audit before I left the facility. I walked out of the office and decided to take the stairs. I pushed the door open to the stairwell and a loud alarm sounded. One nursing assistant came running down the hall, "You have to push the code in on this panel before opening the door. Otherwise, this alarm goes off and we have to worry that a resident is going in here." She didn't appear disheveled or out of breath and her genuine care and concern struck me as a person with exceptional integrity.

I trudged up the filthy stairwell and into the second floor where the alarms once again sounded. This time, there were no staff members available to rush to this door alarm. I pushed the code that was given to me and proceeded to the nurse pushing a medicine cart.

"Good afternoon. My name is Dr. Wellington and I'm the new facility administrator. May I have access to your BGM book (blood glucose monitoring book) please," I said.   "Listen, I'm really swamped. Do you mind getting it yourself? It's on the nursing station," she replied in a squeaky voice.

"That's not a problem. I'll get it from the station and review it. Thanks!"

The nursing station was no easy task to navigate. Papers were piled on top of papers. The sea of binders all had handwritten identifiers on the spines. Many of these were hard to read because of the age of the binder. Once I located the binder, I opened it up and began reviewing, '*Blood Glucose 345, Insulin Units Administered 4, Follow-Up BG 170*'. Then I looked at the parameters and physician orders and they indicated that any blood glucose reading from '*300 – 350, administer 6 units of regular*'. Not only did the nurse fail to follow the physician's order, the resident's blood glucose level did not return to a normal level.

I turned the page of the flimsy black binder to see another mistake and yet another and yet another. Then, I reached over to the fax machine, opened the drawer and pulled a blank sheet of paper out. Immediately, I started a full audit of all the mistakes. In the morning, I would meet with the Director of Nursing to discuss these errors and the need to start re-education of the nursing personnel and continuous quality monitoring.

The audit, however, took me six hours. I audited the entire building's BGM books to learn that the facility had done nothing to fix the initial problem. I wondered what the corporate nurse, Latisha Howard, was actually doing when she arrived at this property. Losing track of time, I realized I needed to stop when my yawns became unbearable.

I put the audit on the administrator's desk, turned off the lights and closed the door as I exited. I buttoned my coat and felt the wetness under my arms. I forgot to remove the coat when I started the audits and didn't realize how much I sweat. The lobby door slid to the side and I walked out of the facility into the cold. It was snowing and the lights from the building were glaring on the snow. It was peaceful.

Day 2

"Good morning, team," I said as I introduced myself in the first morning meeting that I was to run in this facility. The conference room was a barren room with no wall decorations, white painted walls, and three tables put together from the dining room to form some resemblance of a conference room table. When I spoke out loud, the room echoed.

Being the day after Christmas, I expected only a part of the team to arrive. That was not the case today. Since the building was in such poor condition, not a single member of the department manager team was permitted to take any additional time away from the building. The conference room was packed with fourteen people, each a director of their respective departments.

As the room went in a circle introducing themselves to me, the one person I wanted to speak with the most was not in the room. The Director of Nursing arrived twenty minutes after the meeting started wearing black jeans, a see through satin top that showed her bra underneath, and her hair up in braids. "Well, good morning. I'm Dr. Wellington the new administrator."

"I know who you are. Just so you know there is no way I can get here by 9 for this meeting. I suggest we move it to 9:30."

"We can discuss that later but for now the meeting will be at 9 and you'll be expected to arrive on time. What is your name?" She looked at me in disgust, put a grin on her face, and pulled out her iPhone and began text messaging. "And, you'll need to put that away when we're in a meeting."

She slowly put her iPhone on the table, exposing her professionally designed nails, and rolled her eyes. "Okay, Dr. Wellington. Whatever you say." Her tone mocked me.

"And, what is your name?"

"I'm LaToya Williams the Director of Nursing here," she said smugly. "And, before you go blaming this shit on me, you better have a conversation with Shmuey. I came here six months ago as a favor to him."

"Okay, why don't we sit down and talk after this meeting," and then I turned to the team and continued, "but I want everyone to know that I started reviewing our statement of deficiencies and conducted an audit yesterday. We do have issues but I think we can get through these if we structure the facility correctly and hold ourselves accountable. We'll get there team. Now, let's talk about the census."

The meeting proceeded without any further interruptions or problems. On several occasions, I glanced towards LaToya to see her staring at me. Her breathing was intense and she pursed her lips tightly. She appeared to be getting angrier as each minute passed. When the meeting was over, I picked up my legal pad and stood up to leave. "You know what, you will not disrespect me in front of anyone again. You got that Mr. Man," said LaToya.

"Let's go to my office and talk about this," I responded. She followed me with very intense movements talking under her breath the entire time. She mumbled, '*This motherfucker thinks hes tough. We gonna handle this shit.*'

We walked into the still filthy administrator's office and I instructed her to have a seat at the conference table. She pulled the chair from the table with great force. I turned around and shut the door as quietly as possible so as not to agitate her any further.

I sat down across the table from her and opened, "I'm not sure what that was all about in the conference room but what I am sure about is how uncomfortable everyone in that room felt. Are you intimidated by me?"

"Intimidated by you? I am never intimidated by white men. You put me on blast in front of everyone. The only reason I came to this office was for an apology," she responded.

"Okay, first and foremost, we're not going to use race as any bargaining tools in this facility. Secondly, I cannot see how you were put 'on blast'. And, I'm not issuing you an apology. You barged into the meeting twenty minutes late, justified your lateness, and demanded that the time be changed to fit your schedule without even thinking about the welfare of this team."

LaToya looked over at me and grinned. "You think you got this on lockdown? Wait until Shmuey gets here. We'll see who's in charge then." Then, she stood up and started for the door.

I raised my now deepening voice, "I'm not done. Sit down." She looked at me and continued towards the door. "I said sit down now." She turned around and sighed loudly and marched back to the table, yanking a chair at full force and then plopping down into the chair like a small child.

"You have apparently had some traumatic experiences here I this building. I am not the person that has treated you poorly. We have a lot of work to get done in this building and I just don't see why you are so disgruntled when so much of this falls on your shoulders."

"You see, that is what pisses me off. Everyone thinks this is my fault. It's not my fault." Her eyes now welled up with tears. She was an experienced manipulator. The angry tone to the sad flip was something she had used many times and I was not an inexperienced administrator. After all, I once worked in clinical social work.

I reached for the box of tissue on the table and slid it over to her. She grabbed three tissues and blew her nose with it. She never used the tissue to wipe her eyes. "You know what, let's end this for now. Why don't you head back to you office and we'll meet later to discuss the deficiencies and an action plan to get this building back to compliance." She stood up patiently and without force, opened the office door slowly, and walked out without any mumbling. LaToya thought she had me fooled. She was wrong.

Moments later, Jane knocked on the open door. She wore a conservative ensemble of purple and black with high heels. Her trademark hanging reading glasses rested on her bosom and her jet black hair was up in a wild bun in the back of her head. "Dr. Wellington, my name is Jane and I'm the receptionist and administrative assistant. If there is ever anything you need, please do let me know. I pretty much handle your schedule and anything else you need."

"Thank you, Jane. As a matter of fact there is one thing and I hope it isn't too demeaning to ask about. Where can I find the coffee?" She smiled and said, "Of course, sir. The coffee can be found in the executive lounge across the hall. But, if you want my advice, I'd say let me go out and get you Starbucks because that coffee is horrible."

"You would actually do that for me?"

"Of course I would. When I step away from the desk, Mary in human resources covers for me. Starbucks is only a few blocks away. Let me do that for you right away. If possible, I'd like to sit down with you to discuss your expectations for an executive assistant and what it is that you will need from me. I'm looking forward to working with you and I have heard great things."

'*How has she heard anything about me?*' I wondered. This building was turning out to be just as fun as reading the mountain of paper that was their statement of deficiencies from the health department.

"Before you leave, would you mind notifying housekeeping that this office needs to be cleaned."

"Right away sir."

Moments later, I heard commotion coming from the main lobby. I walked out to see an ambulance driver holding a plastic garbage bag of clothing and telling someone that they needed to get into the ambulance. "I'm not leaving here. This is my home," came a meek voice from the lady, "You're not throwing me out."

I notice LaToya standing next to her, "You are leaving this facility. We can no longer meet your needs. Besides, you'll like the other facility. It has crazy folks just like you there." Her sarcasm was not lost on this patient. "You'll never get away with this, you bitch," the patient said.

"Ladies, I don't have all day. Can you both book a time for the mud ring later? I have a scheduled to keep," the ambulance driver said as I walked into the lobby.

"What is going on here?" I inquired. "This patient was involuntarily discharged and today is her day to leave."

"Do we have the paperwork for this involuntary discharge somewhere so that we can give it to her?"

"We'll send another copy to her later."

I turned to the patient and asked her for her name, "May I have your name and I give you my word that I will contact you when you get to the other facility?" And, her response was, "Fuck you. You're throwing me out against my will!"

At that moment, the social worker came to the lobby and met with the resident privately. I was unable to hear what she said to her, or any part of the conversation for that matter, but the resident began crying. Latrice, the social worker, cried with her. Then, the resident got into the ambulance and I never heard from her again.

I turned to LaToya, "I want to see a copy of that involuntary discharge document." She replied to me, "There isn't a document. That bitch has been causing us problems since she got here. We just sent her to a psychiatric nursing home and they can deal with her crazy ass."

"LaToya, we can't do that. She has rights!"

"If you don't like what I'm doing, sue me," she said walking away. I made a mental note to report this to the corporate office.

Later that day, after woofing down a peanut butter and jelly sandwich in my now clean but disorganized office, I asked Jane to call the clinical members of the team to my office. This included: Director of Nursing, Assistant Director of Nursing, Restorative Nurse, Rehabilitation Director, and Social Worker. When they arrived, I passed out the packets containing my action plan for this facility – one in which I stayed awake most of the evening creating.

"Ladies, as you know we have very little time to clear this facility before it is decertified. There are a lot of residents and a lot of jobs on the line here and we can't risk making any mistakes. Thus, what you hold in your hands is an action plan. I have also included an audit of the blood glucose monitoring books to determine what progress we have made on the cited deficiency."

"Wait a minute," said LaToya, "you audited my work?"

"That is correct."

"There is like seven sheets of errors in this packet."

"That is correct."

"These people are idiots. You'll find that out as you spend time here." She turned to the restorative nurse, Lashawna, and directed her, "Get on the floors and correct these numbers after this meeting."

Immediately and without thinking about tact I said, "Absolutely not. You will do no such thing. These errors have been made. You can't just go back and correct them on paper. And, as long as I am here we will do things above board. Period. Now that audit is meant to serve as an initial audit. You will retrain the staff on looking at the orders before administering medication and then you will re-audit five times per week a minimum of twenty records. The state health department will then see that we have made progress. We will not falsify documentation under my watch. Do you understand me?"

"Jesus Christ! He doesn't get it. These people are not going to change."

"Well, LaToya, you have been here six months. What exactly have you done to encourage and help them change? Let's talk about that for a moment. All of you in here are going to start managing your departments with integrity and dignity. When your staff see you cut corners, they have no vested interest to get things done right, either. You are responsible for self-accountability and then holding your teams accountable. And, that is exactly what you all will do. Because if you don't, I will hold you accountable."

The room fell silent. And, then the social worker Latrice spoke up and said, "Are you saying you planning on firing us?" I looked at her with bewilderment. This group truly didn't understand what they were up against. "Latrice, this isn't about you getting fired or not. If we don't clear this building in three weeks time, no one here will have a job. The building will close and the residents will be displaced and everyone in this building will be, I repeat, without a job."

Latrice clicked her pen repeatedly after she heard this. She nodded her head from side to side and sighed. "My baby daddy don't pay child support. I can't afford to be without a job. How can we save this building?"

"We're going to start by opening this action plan and getting rolling. And, we're not going to do anything that will jeopardize the integrity of this facility or ourselves. If the surveyors, for one minute, think you are trying to scam them they will not clear this building. We can do this together but I need the team on my side."

The team spent the meeting mostly complaining that they could not manage their direct reports and that they didn't see how they would be successful. One thing struck me as consistent. I would have to fix this building as a solo act if I wanted it to be done right and with integrity. And that, unfortunately, is not realistic in a building that was so large.

At 4pm, I dialed the intercom button and asked Jane to page the department head team to my office. "I'm sorry sir, they all have left."

"What do you mean they all left? They didn't get into the facility until 9 and now they are leaving at 4? Is this a typical day or merely because the holiday is here?"

"This is the schedule every day. If you would like, I will call specific managers' mobile phones and communicate a message. Should I do that?"

"No. That won't be necessary. Thank you, Jane."

I unbuttoned the cuffs on my shirt and rolled the sleeves up to my mid-forearm. Then, I picked up the notepad I had been writing in all day, a copy of the action plan, and a pen and left my office intent on going to the second floor.

The elevator ride was not much fun and the smell, as the day before, was horrendous when I exited the elevator door to the second floor. As was the day before, the residents appeared to have been neglected all day long with poor hygiene and filthy clothing and there was one nurse viewable from the hall.

I walked down to the nurse and asked, "I need to see the TARs (treatment administration records). Where are those located?" She responded, "They are at the nursing station."

I thank her and walked back towards the nursing station and sat down. The sea of binders had not magically organized overnight. The BGM book, however, was laying flat on the desk. Instead of grabbing the TARs, I decided to open the BGM to see if there were any changes this day with nurses following the physicians' orders.

"Unbelievable," I said out loud. No one was within earshot, thankfully. The 'errors' that I discovered yesterday were all crossed out and marked '*error*' and a new number inserted. Each page had many of these markings and all with the same initials on the side of them, '*LW*'. LaToya went through the book and falsified the records even after I instructed her to not do this.

I removed the pages to the entire binder and photocopied them using the fax machine on the desk. The machine scanned and printed slowly and produced a heating element smell. It was nauseating. Once done, I collected the copies and placed the originals back into the binder.

After returning downstairs, I jotted a note to myself:

> *In the morning, I will need to meet with the corporate office and terminate LaToya for falsification of records and altering licensed nursing professionals' documentation. Then, I will need to file a report with the state department of licensing against her nursing license. This is a high priority.*

Then, I turned to the computer and proceeded to type an email to Shmuey:

We have a serious problem here at the facility with the Director of Nursing, LaToya. She bullies the team, shows up late to meetings, slams doors, threatens me, and now she is falsifying documentation. I would like to make a change and quickly. Let's meet offsite to discuss this in more detail tomorrow. This cannot wait.

I hit the 'send' button and turned around to the desk. It wasn't as much of a mess as it was this morning but it certainly was a problem. I organized piles into 'before Joseph' and 'current'. Then, I turned to the computer to turn it off. Shmuey had already responded.

Shmuey's response was brief:

Let's meet at Appelbees at Noon three blocks from the facility. I can't eat there but at least we can have a drink. I'll see you then.

It was astounding. He wanted to 'have a drink' at Noon when I would have to return to the office. This day wasn't getting any better for me.

A knock on the door caught my attention. "Dr. Wellington, I'm leaving for the day. Is there anything I can do for you before I leave," Jane asked politely. "No. Thank you for checking in with me. I think I'm heading out for the night, too. Have a great night," I said. "You too, sir."

The shiny black briefcase I brought with me this morning was sitting underneath the desk. There was no way I was working at home this evening. I was exhausted. I grabbed my coat and said out loud to myself, "Tomorrow ought to be a real doosy."

At least, the air outside was refreshing. It was cold, crisp, and clean. Even the white snow brought serenity to a mind that was filled with anxiety and exhaustion. Inside the facility was a dense fog of pressure and toxicity. I debated whether or not to return to this facility tomorrow. '*You must return because the people here need you. You, at least, are able to leave in the evening*,' resounded in my mind's conscience. I would need rest. I drove away, stopped at Taco Bell for a Quesadilla, and went home to sleep.

Day 3

The echoes in the conference room bludgeoned my ears. When one member of the team talked, it wasn't so bad. This team, however, didn't understand that they should take turns speaking. Each person got louder as the next person got louder.

Loudly, I said, "Enough. Let's get this started." And, my own voice ricocheted back into my ears while my head pounded even harder. "Sheesh, you don't have to yell at us," said the activity director.

"Dr. Wellington, do you have any idea what happened yesterday?"

"This is a real mess."

"I can't believe this is happening to us now of all times."

"She died and we fucked up. Someone is going to jail over this."

I intervened because the comments were coming too fast. "What is everyone talking about?"

LaShawna was the first to speak up. "Diane on the Unit 2D died yesterday. Didn't anyone call you?"

"Not to sound unconcerned but why would anyone call me for a resident death?"

"Dr. Wellington, you don't understand. When she left the downstairs dialysis department, she was bleeding. They didn't apply the clamps after treatment."

"Please tell me you are joking," I said as my head pounded even harder now. The throbbing wouldn't subside even after two cups of coffee and two Advil.

LaShawna continued, "When she got upstairs, she sat next to the nursing station and by the time the nurse found her, the entire floor was soaked with blood."

I sprung into action. "I want the clinical interdisciplinary team to stay behind and everyone else is dismissed with the express understanding that none of this information leaves this room." Some team members picked up their coffee and notepads while others had nothing with them. They left whispering amongst themselves. This was never going to remain a secret and I was, sadly, well aware of that.

"Where is LaToya? It is 9:15am," I said as LaToya barged into the meeting. "Are you asking for me?" she said while standing next to her was Shmuey. She grinned at me with a silent mocking sneer.

"LaToya, were you aware that Diane died last night?"

"Who?"

"You know, your patient Diane on Unit 2?"

"I have no idea who that is," she said antagonistically.

"This is truly a surprise to me. No one called you?"

"Why would they call me?"

"Enough of this. I want a detailed report of what happened. The nurses that worked last night need to be called and I want the entire dialysis department team in my office in twenty minutes. We need written statements. LaToya, please go upstairs and bring the entire hardback chart to me and lock her electronic record from viewing until we have the chance to send this to risk management." Although I wasn't finished with my directives, Shmuey chimed in, "What is going on?"

"There is an allegation that a resident on Unit 2 received dialysis here and that she bled out and died upstairs because we failed to properly clamp her," I responded.

Without missing a beat, and breathing loudly, he responded, "You gotta be fucking kidding me. LaToya let's get that chart right away." And, with that, Shmuey left with LaToya. The team that remained, four in all, remained quiet the entire time that Shmuey was in the room. Once the left, the gossip began.

Latrice mocked Shmuey once he left, "Yeah, LaToya let's go get that chart so we can go to your office and knock them boots off you."

The rest of the team chimed in, "He knows he doesn't give a shit about this building. He just wants to hit that and leave for the day," "She's a hoe and they ain't going to get that chart, best believe that," and other comments. It was disturbing but I refused to allow this to go on any longer, "Folks, we aren't going to engage in this type of conversation while I'm in these meetings. We have a lot of work to get done now."

LaShawna chimed in, "But you don't understand Dr. Wellington. That's why this bitch ain't getting fixed. That hoe don't know shit about what's going on here and she ain't going to review no chart. Watch what happens. Charting going to be missing. Nurses will get fired to protect her hoe ass. Ain't nobody going to say nothing either cause they scared."

"Are you telling me that documentation will come up missing," I asked. "That's exactly what she's saying," said Latrice.

"Let's dismiss for now and we'll regroup later on this afternoon."

I walked into the administrative offices area and saw Jane sitting at her desk. "Good morning, Jane. How are you?" She looked up at me and smiled, "Very good sir. How are you?" I replied, "I've had better days. May I see you for moment?"

Jane walked behind me slowly. Her heels clacked on the floor in a rhythm. "Jane, I need you to write a memo from me and get it posted at the nursing stations."

"Very good sir. Let me get my steno pad and pencil and you can dictate. Just give me a moment."

She left the office and returned within moments. After she sat down at the conference table, "Please begin sir."

"Greetings Team Members. Please be advised that the administrator must be called for any and all situations involving incidents and/or accidents that result in injury, however minor. He should also be notified of any resident deaths, hospitalizations, family disputes, resident behaviors, fire alarms, disasters, staffing issues, or any other unusual occurrence. He may be reached directly at xxx-xxx-xxxx."

"Please allow me to read that back to you sir," and she read the entire sentence back in perfect unison to my brief but powerful memorandum. "That sounds perfect," I said. "I'll get that typed and posted at the nursing stations and by the timeclock right away, sir."

Jane removed her reading glasses, folded them and let them drop onto her bosom with the glasses rope she kept around her neck. She picked up her steno pad and started to walk out of the room when she turned around, "Dr. Wellington, did you have your coffee this morning by chance?"

I giggled like a child. "I had a few cups of coffee. To be honest, I have a horrible headache and the coffee isn't working."

"You wait right here. I have a solution for you," she went to her desk and pulled out a prescription strength Ibuprofen. "If this doesn't cure that headache, nothing will." She handed me a glass of water that she procured from the water cooler outside my office. I quickly swallowed the pill. "There. That should do it," and with that she walked out of the office.

Then, I looked at my watch (I was wearing a stainless steel square Bulova watch that I had received as a gift) and noticed that nearly 30 minutes had passed since I told LaToya to bring me the hardback chart. *This is absolutely unacceptable*, I thought to myself, *and Shmuey should know better, too.*

Instead of waiting, I headed out of my office with the express intent on procuring the chart myself. I needed to be prepared to admit wrongdoing and notify the insurance company or send to risk management to prepare for a battle in the event that one ever came. A battle was certainly brewing either way, and my experienced gut told me something was wrong here.

I walked down the hall and, right before I stepped onto the elevator, I noticed the light to LaToya's office was on with the door shut. The elevator door opened and I turned around and marched towards LaToya's office. I knocked once and pushed the door open. *Gasp!*

LaToya was laying on her desk with her shirt on but her pants off. Shmuey had his erect penis out through the zipper on his pants and was having sex with her right on her desk. He looked disheveled, his pants wrinkled, and his yarmulke still in place. The sweat from his forehead was visible and shiny. He looked at me, "Get the fuck out of here. Don't you know how to fucking knock on the door? Goddammit!"

I closed the door to her office and waited by the elevator once again. The elevator took a few minutes and Shmuey never came out of the office. I wondered if he was taking his time to actually finish what he was doing.

As I waited for the elevator, my mind raced. *There is simply no way that I am going to get that lady out of this building and get someone who knows what they are doing if he's having sex with her. I'm in for a fight here. How in the hell am I going to get this done without the backing of Shmuey and corporate support?* I despaired. The elevator door opened and I walked in and pushed the button for the second floor. I looked around the elevator and made a mental note to have maintenance take a look at all of the wheelchair scratches on the bottom of the elevator walls.

When I got to the second floor, I sent an email from my Blackberry to Sarah Dustfy in human resources:

Sarah, It's Joseph Wellington. We need to talk. It's urgent. Please call me. Thank you. Dr. W.

The smell on this floor was pungent and striking once again. The nursing station was in the same disarray as usual. I looked on the chart rack and found Diane's hardback chart and pulled it. "Hey, you can't just take a chart. Make sure you sign it out," came a voice from a distance away.

A very short black woman was charging very fast towards me. "I know you are the administrator and all but these are my records if you know what I mean," she said. "Um, your records?" I asked.

"I'm Sharice in medical records and I'm sorry to be so rude but I can't seem to keep the records straight when everyone takes them without signing them out."

"That's completely understandable, no worries. I'm Dr. Wellington. Where is the clip board to sign these out? I'm going to hold on to this chart for a few days."

"A few days?" she said in disbelief while raising her voice an octave. "That resident has expired and I don't have long to close the chart."

"Not a problem. As soon as I have finished with this, I will be sure to notify you. No worries."

Sharice smiled, "Okay, you're the boss." Then, she proceeded back down the hall. I watched her walk for a few moments while the lights flickered. She disappeared into the last room before the emergency stairwell. If I remembered correctly, she just walked into the activity director's office and not her medical records office.

I turned around and, holding the chart, proceeded back to the elevator. I pushed the button repeatedly to make sure that the elevator button light came on. It illuminated after several pushes. "Nothing in this damn place works," I said out loud without realizing I was audible with frustration.

"You got that right sugar," said a resident next to the elevator in a wheelchair. "Oh, my goodness. I should never have said that out loud. I do apologize." A quick review of her appearance worried me – she wore a hospital gown, clearly had not been showered in a long time, and was not wearing shoes. In her hand, she held a rosary and smiled at me.

"Don't apologize for speaking the truth. I just hope that you can fix this," she said. As much as I wanted to stay and talk with her, the strong smell of urine coming from her was offensive. The elevator door opened, "I'm going to do my best. What is your name sweetheart," I asked. "It is Evelyn. Everyone up here calls me Evvy, though." I then said, "It is nice to meet you Evvy. I'm on it and will see you soon."

My heart ached for what I saw and I thought silently, '*A part of me hopes that this facility gets shuttered. This is no way for anyone to live.*' I was overcome with sadness. Before I could do any additional thinking to myself, the elevator doors opened to a much more palatable scene. These two floors were night and day.

I glanced over to LaToya's office and noticed that the door was wide open and the lights were off. I strolled near and peered inside. LaToya's purse was gone, too.

When I finally arrived to the administrative office area, Jane stopped me, "Dr. Wellington, Shmuey wanted me to tell you that he was taking LaToya to breakfast and that he will meet with you at Noon at Applebees."

"Thank you for Jane. Did LaToya seem okay when she left with him? Is she coming back?"

"Dr. Wellington, may I speak with you in your office for a moment?" she looked worried. "Of course. Come on in," I reassured her as we walked into my office. She closed the door behind her and looked through the corners of the glass as if she was watching for someone.

"Dr. Wellington, I am not a gossip but there is something you should know. Shmuey and LaToya have been having an affair for the past six months. He protects her. Every administrator has been fired after they complained about her. You need to know that because the rumor here is that you are going to get fired because you challenged her during a meeting. I really like you and I'm worried about you. Please be careful."

Jane was genuinely worried. I could see the concern in her eyes and hear the motherly tone in her voice.

"Thank you, Jane. I'll definitely take that advice. My job has become more complicated because of that situation. We'll get it done but it's going to be more difficult," I sighed with exhaustion.

"Great. Now, I hear your wife's birthday is June 8th. Is that true?"

"Huh? Have you been conducting a background check on us?" I laughed inquisitively. "No. She called and told me her birthday when I asked her. I have marked it in the calendar and will double check with you when we get closer for the gift I should pick up. And, don't worry about a thing. I'll get flowers sent to her office for Valentines Day and all the major holidays."

"Whoa! Gee, thanks Jane. You are amazing. I'll have to return the favor," I smiled, "Meanwhile, do you know the telephone number to the risk management department?"

"I don't think the company has a risk management department. I can give you the cell phone number to the regional nurse consultant. Her name is Latisha Howard. Let me get her on the phone for you."

"Thank you very much."

Latisha, however, never answered her telephone and I left a voicemail, "*Hello Latisha. This is Joseph Wellington. I have a file that needs to be assessed for risk management purposes and an investigation opened. Please call me at the facility as soon as you get this message. Thanks.*"

She never did call me back.

I waited at the Applebees for over an hour for Shmuey to arrive, without any return calls from his mobile telephone. Finally, at 1pm, I paid for my Coca-Cola and headed back to the facility.

"Good afternoon, Dr. Wellington," Mary said while sitting at the front desk. "Hello there. Where is Jane," I asked. "Jane is on lunch and I usually sit in for her when she goes on lunch."

Shaking the snow off of my shoes by the front door, I proceeded to talk across the room, "Did Shmuey get back yet?"

"Let me check for you," she said. I don't see him checked back in, "Nope. It looks like LaToya is still out so Shmuey is definitely not back yet." She smiled and laughed a little.

"What does that have to do with anything?"

"Oh, come on. You hold a doctorate. There's certainly got to be some intelligence in there," she said sarcastically. "Did Latisha ring for me while I was out?"

"Sorry, Dr. Wellington. I don't have any telephone calls for you. I can check your box for you if you like." I replied, "That won't be necessary. Can you please page Sharice to my office? Thanks!"

The snow was finally off of my shoes. They were still wet, though. After slipping on the plastic runner, I decided to walk on the carpeting. *Replace the carpet during Spring*, I made a mental note.

I hung up my coat and scarf and Sharice walked into the office. "What can I do for you?" she asked in a strong tone. "I don't want to beat about the bush. I need to know how to lock an electronic record so that only a few people with passwords can access a specific file."

"Oh, that is easy. Let me show you," as she walked over to my desk and clicked a program on the computer. "You have to follow these steps," and proceeded to give me information.

"Hmmm, that is strange. This file was locked and then unlocked. There is a lot of documentation here that has been deleted. Just give me a minute. Let me open the full access viewing on this charting."

"What do you mean 'full access viewing' on this chart?"

"It means that all data that has been keyed into this chart will show regardless of whether it has been listed as an error or fully deleted."

"Why would anyone want to delete any charting at all? Couldn't they just error it out if they made a mistake?"

"They certainly could do so. Give me a minute here."

She pushed some keys, played with the mouse, and clicked several items. Then she clicked 'search' and all of the deleted charting appeared for all departments. All charting for Diane had been deleted four hours prior. Sharice proclaimed with authority, "It looks like LaToya has deleted all charting for the past forty-eight hours for all departments for the expired resident."

"How do you know it was LaToya?"

"Every action anyone in here does is recorded. Let me show you," and she pointed to the section that shows who did what action. "LaToya Williams is listed under all of the deletions."

"Please print out all of those pages for me. Also, you moved really fast so I couldn't get all of the steps. Can you show me again how you were able to pull all of that information up?"

"Sure."

Later that day, Shmuey and LaToya arrived to the facility. It was 3:45pm. Shmuey walked into the office and told me that LaToya was heading home for the day.

"Shmuey, I'm a very direct person so let me be direct with you. What you are doing is causing a serious problem in this facility. By you sleeping with her, it is causing the facility to not run properly. The building is on the road to closure without her help and you took her out all day. That is not helpful."

"Joseph, you are really getting on my nerves. We all fuck our staff and you know god damn well that we do. So get off your fucking pedestal you jackass."

"Fine. If you don't want to hear it in the nicest way I was able to deliver it, then hear this. When LaToya walks into this building tomorrow morning, I will be issuing her termination along with filing a formal report against her professional license for altering patient records and falsifying documentation. I haven't decided whether or not to file a criminal case. And, you will see a filing on your professional license as an accomplice. Get that woman out of this facility and I *might not* take that action. I won't ask again."

Shmuey sat down in a conference table chair, still wearing his coat and put his black fedora on the table, and folded his hands. He pursed his lips and squeezed them. Then he moved them upwards in his thinking position. He unfolded his hands and then grabbed his yarmulke and moved it around a few times on his head. With a deep breath in, he looked directly at me, "If I move her to another building, will you back off?"

I lowered my eyebrows tensely, "That depends. Are you going to have another director of nursing in this building by 8am? And, will you consider terminating her to avoid further risk management to this company?"

"Joseph, you and I both know I can't fire her. If I do, she's got too much shit on me."

"You're kidding," I responded sarcastically.

"Don't fucking push me. You're asking me to fire the chick I'm nailing so you can look good. Let me talk to Joseph and see if I can move her to a smaller facility."

"Shmuey, let me tell you something. Do you know anything about the Catholic Church and how they moved around priests? She may not be molesting people but she is causing a great deal of pain and suffering to patients and staff by what she is doing. You can't just bounce her from facility to facility to protect her. Ultimately, this will cause pain to this organization's bottom line. Mark my words."

"Fine. I'll make a decision. Look for an email tonight with your new director of nursing. Now, can we talk about this damn survey before I leave?"

My body tension released and I decided I wasn't interested in the fight. The light was fading outside at such an early hour and I wanted to get some work done. "Sure. I have put together an action plan….."

He interrupted me with sarcasm and rolling eyes, "I'm sure you did a great job with your action plan but I'm going to pay the surveyors. We don't have enough time to clear this survey. Once I pay them, do you think you can stabilize this facility enough so that we can get it sold?"

"I already told you I don't want any connection with you bribing a surveyor. If you do that, please leave me out of it. As for getting this building sold, I wasn't aware that this was the direction but I can get it ready for sale. That's not a problem."

"Good," he said looking at me with a smile, "now keep the LaToya stuff a secret for both of us and we'll get along just fine."

"Shmuey, I don't give a damn about your affairs. Just get me a new director of nursing by tomorrow morning." He smiled and stood up, his coat still on, put his fedora on his head, and walked out of the office door.

I sat down at the desk and looked out the window. He walked to his gray Lexus SUV and opened the door. The roof light inside the car went on and I saw another person sitting in the passenger seat of his car. I now knew why LaToya and him arrived at the same time.

The light was fading fast outside. The documents that were printed sat on my desk. Instead of putting them to the side, I packed them into my briefcase under the desk. I wrote a post-it note '*photocopy entire file*' and placed it on Diane's hardback chart.

Then, Jane knocked on my door ever so slightly, "Dr. Wellington, if you don't mind I'm planning on leaving a little early today. I need to pick up my granddaughter from day care."

"That's not a problem. How old is your granddaughter?"

"She is four. You want to see pictures?" she said as her face lit up with excitement.

"That would be great. Before you leave, though, would you page housekeeping to spray something in this office. There is a horrible body odor smell that I don't want to linger in here all night. I also need to speak with the clinical team members."

"Very good sir. I'll take care of it right away. I alerted the team this morning that you wanted them to stay later than 4pm and they all waited around. Let me get the pictures for you. You'll find her adorable."

Her granddaughter's pictures were absolutely adorable. She had the cutest little blonde locks of hair that so many children have and chubby cheeks. Jane was a proud grandma that beamed from ear to ear when she heard me say how cute her granddaughter was.

Jane looked up and acknowledged, "The team is here, Dr. Wellington. I'm going to head out. You have a great night." "You too, Jane," I replied. Each one of them was holding a coat and a purse. They were ready to leave the building.

"Everyone, please take a seat," I said. "Now that the day is over and a few changes have been made, we're going to talk about my expectations. Tomorrow morning, a new director of nursing starts in this facility."

LaShawna responded in disbelief, "You think you got that bitch out of here?"

"LaShawna, we won't refer to anyone in that tone in my meetings but to answer your question, yes she is now gone. The new DON will start tomorrow. And, before anyone asks I don't know who the appointed individual is."

Everyone looked around and talked amongst each other. The administrator's office had carpeting and the noise didn't ricochet like the conference room. "Now that I have given you a moment to let that sink in, let's talk about my expectations going forward."

"First and foremost, I want everyone here in this building at 7:30am for the first meeting we will call 'Stand Up' and no one is able to leave this building until 5pm when we will have a last meeting of the day called 'Step Down'. Will that be a problem?" There were no responses from the conference table. No one nodded their heads, even. "These meetings will provide the 'action plan for the day' and the 'report of progress for the day.'"

"Next, each of you will be responsible to audit your teams' work and productivity. No one is permitted to alter, falsify, or adjust any paperwork in this facility. That includes in the computer system. We do not 'fix' paperwork. We make the amendments to these documents only if it was our work and leave the original information in there. Can anyone tell me why I am saying this? Why is this so important to me?"

Latrice spoke up first, "It's like you said. You don't want our integrity questioned. And, um, duh!" She was sarcastic but supportive.

"Next item, you will all start training your staff and holding them accountable for the training expectations. And, all of you are required to be on the clinical floors throughout the day. This doesn't mean you have to be out of your office all day but take turns. The second floor is not fit for a dog kennel and I am ashamed of it."

Then, the team chimed in with: "We can't be on the floor if we have all of this paperwork that is due," and "There is no way I can be on the floor," and "How can you ask us to do more work than we are already doing," and "We can barely get our jobs done now." The tension in the room grew by the ever-lengthening second.

"Let me tell you folks a quick story. There was a home that I once worked at that had many deficiencies. That home struggled with their director of nursing and the bullying. The state arrived and didn't approve the plan of correction and continued the citations. Then, the staff refused to help out on the floor. The facility was decertified. Now, none of the staff had anything to complain about because they had no work. The building closed down and all the jobs were lost. Does this sound familiar?"

"Yes, it does," said Patricia. Patricia was the therapy director that had, until this minute, been quiet. She was highly intimidated by the director of nursing – even though she held a doctorate in physical therapy. "That sounds like us."

"That is correct, Patricia. That is because that is the story I will have to tell at my next facility if we don't get this fixed and that means we are all going to have to put in long hours – probably longer than 5pm – and really get dug in here. I know you all love it here and are loyal. So, let's not let this building fail."

"You sound like Sister Mary Clarence," joked LaShawna. I provided a perplexed look. "Like Sister Act the movie? Oh, come on you can't tell me you ain't seen that movie!" Then, everyone laughed.

"I'm adding that to my list of movies to watch this weekend. Next, everyone will need to listen to me very closely to make this happen. Please don't be afraid to disagree but don't hold too tightly to your opinions because not all of our opinions and decisions will be the best way to do things."

"If that bitch in the DON office would have been that way, we wouldn't be in this mess," said Patricia. I stared at the table for a moment. Everyone turned to Patricia in disbelief that she would speak with profanity. "All of you were thinking the same thing so don't look at me like that."

"Lastly, everyone in this room will operate with integrity. There will be no lying, deceit, manipulation, usury, or anything below board. We will make this happen because we can make this a success the right way. The residents will appreciate it, the families will appreciate it, you will go home at night feeling great about yourselves, and the state survey teams will appreciate it. I have faith this is possible."

Latrice smiled and looked as if she was about to cry. "You are so real, Dr. Wellington, and I'm so glad you came. Ya'll let's make up with each other before we leave because LaToya pinned each one of us against each other and it ain't right. We need to let go of what has happened in the past."

Strangely, the team stood up and hugged each other. This team needed more than a facility turnaround. They needed the toxicity to leave the building so that they could heal. It was too soon to tell whether or not this would be good enough. Only time would provide me with the information I needed.

After everyone left, I closed the blinds to the office and sat down at the desk and wrote:

Although the DON will be reassigned and a new DON brought to the facility, as promised by Shmuey, I am required to report this to the state department of health and the state professional licensing agency. I will do this within twenty-four hours because I have no choice. In the morning, I need to create an action plan to ensure this never happens again in the hope that the state doesn't provide me with any additional deficiencies that I won't be able to clear in time before decertification. Also, I will need to report LaToya's license even though I made the agreement with Shmuey. I will need to pull LaToya's file in the morning from human resources.

Sidenote: Pull Sharice's file for review. She seems undervalued here.

Then, I put that entire notepad with that information into my briefcase along with several other items, including spreadsheets that I created for plan of correction audits. I was confident that tomorrow would be a better day for a great starting point.

I put on my coat, a black fedora, and black leather gloves. I reached for the briefcase and strapped it over my shoulder and then left the office.

When I reached the lobby, I heard a young girl's voice say, "Have a great night, Dr. Wellington." The young girl was sitting at the receptionist desk and waving. She was skinny with long brown hair and wearing a sweater that was far too revealing for a young girl her age.

"Thank you very much. What is your name?"

"I am Sandra, the evening receptionist," she said.

"It is lovely to meet you Sandra. You also have a wonderful night. Be careful driving. The snow is supposed to come down pretty heavy later this evening."

I walked outside and felt the cold air once again. The air was exhilarating. This day was one of great success. I walked to the car, put my briefcase in the back seat, and sat down in the drivers seat. Instead of turning on the car, I stared at myself in the mirror for a moment and was reminded that I was no longer young. I took a deep breath, started the car, and drove away.

Day 4

"Good morning Mary," I said, "I need to see the files for Sharice and LaToya please." It was 7am and Mary had already arrived to the facility. Jane mentioned that Mary usually arrived earlier than anyone else and, often, stayed later than everyone else. "Is there a reason, Dr. Wellington?" she asked.

I took a sip of my Starbucks Caramel Macchiato, which was still piping hot. "LaToya no longer works here and I'd like to get some information from her file to finalize a report. And, I am really impressed with Sharice. I'd like to see her salary and her background to see if there is anything we are missing that we could do better." Mary reached into her desk drawer and pulled out a chain with four keys attached. She selected the correct key, walked over to the file cabinet marked, Current Employees, and unlocked the top lock.

After she pulled open two drawers and selected the files, she said, "Here you are Dr. Wellington. If there is anything else I can do for you, please don't hesitate to let me know." I proceeded to exit her office when she said, "Dr. Wellington, not to sound rude but you should know a few things about Sharice. She may seem nice to you but she is rude to everyone else. Staff members have actually lost their jobs after threatening to meet her in the parking lot. She is not the person you think she is."

"Thanks for the information. Before I leave, is this all of the information in their human resources files?" I asked. Mary looked up at the ceiling for a moment, sighed, and responded sarcastically, "Of course not. Let me dash through the rose garden in the main courtyard and pull the rest from the west wing." I laughed hysterically. I used my sleeve to wipe the tears from my eyes. Then, she laughed. I felt a mutual respect develop in that moment.

"Okay, I got it, I got it. Thanks," I said. When I exited her office, I noticed Patricia, the therapy director, walking into a side door. "Good morning, Patricia. How are you?"

"Good morning, Dr. Wellington. You are here early. How are you?"

"I'm doing well. I didn't think anyone else arrived this early."

"If I don't arrive this early, I don't get my work finished. So, I hide out in the therapy gym office so no one can reach me. That way, I get things accomplished and everyone is happy. That includes me." She winked at me and proceeded into the therapy gym doors. Tempted to follow her, I got to the therapy gym doors and turned around. If she didn't want to be bothered, she meant by anyone and that included me.

I walked to my office and sat back down with my coffee. The files were the thinnest I had ever seen for a human resources file. LaToya's file held four documents: Resume with a coffee cup stain on it, Signature for Keys, and Federal and State Withholding forms with a signature that was barely legible. There was nothing else. It was as if the file had been thinned before I was able to get to it. But, it had the most important information I needed to know – her social security number and her professional license number.

Next, I looked at Sharice's file. This file had the exact same information in it. There was nothing in terms of training on abuse and neglect, resident behaviors, company policy and procedure review, or anything else that mattered. *Where are all the documents that are required?* I wondered. Then, something caught my eye. Sharice held an MBA from Harvard University. *Why in the world is she working as medical records clerk with this educational background?*

I called Sharice's office at 8:30am and asked her to come to my office and collect Diane's record. I would need a photocopy of the entire chart and asked her to print a hard copy of the entire record inside the computer system. "Afterwards, I will need you to collect the medication records and treatment records from the floor and have them photocopied and placed in the same file for me. If there are any other records for Diane anywhere else, please collect those and photocopy them for me, too. You may have the file back once you are done."

"Anything else you need from me? How about I come over to your house and scrub your floors?" Sharice was in a bad mood. At first, I thought she was joking and cracked a smile. "What? You think that is funny? I have my own stuff to do and now you are making me run errands because that airhead in the nursing office screwed you over."

"Sharice, only the clinical team members are aware of this. It is not public news yet, apparently. LaToya no longer works here."

"Hallelujah!"

Now, I smiled. "But, we have a lot of work to do to undo the damage she caused and I'm going to need a lot of help from your department. Are you with me here?"

"You bet your ass I'm with you!" She turned on her right heel and marched out of the room with the chart in her arms. The chart looked large because of her height and size.

I looked down at the desk and started my list of priorities for the day. "Dr. Wellington, we need to see you right away," came a voice from the door to the office. I looked up and saw a nurse standing in the doorway. "What is going on?" I responded.

"Gerald, a patient in 2C, says that the maintenance man threatened him and he is afraid to come out of his room." She was erratic and trying to excite me. I had seen this behavior before amongst nursing home personnel.

"Did you ask Gerald to give you a detailed explanation and did you write out a statement? Was there anyone else involved? Is the maintenance man still here? Who is the maintenance man?"

"Um, can you start those questions over," she responded. I stood up from the desk and started walking towards her, "Let's just go meet with Mr. Gerald right now. You'll need to write a statement for me of what he said to you." She never responded to me. Instead she led me to the elevator and pushed the call button for me.

On the elevator ride up I asked, "What is your name?"

"I'm Lois. I work the morning shift."

"It is nice to meet you, Lois."

Her uniform was neat, clean, and pressed. She took very good care of her hygiene and she smelled good. Her hair was up in a large clip in the back of her head with many pieces all over the place. I wondered if she was a newer nurse.

We stepped off of the elevator and the smell of fresh paint was overwhelming. Down the hall in front of the elevator was a man painting with a roller on a large wooden handle. He was already a mess with green paint on his clothing and white specks of dust all over his hair at this early hour.

"Gerald's room is right down this way. Be prepared. He has not had his methadone yet and, even though he is frightened, he can get a little grumpy," came a forewarning from her. A man was painting in the other hallway and yet this hallway still had flickering lights. We knocked on Gerald's door and heard, "Come in" come from the other side.

I turned the dirty doorknob, pushed the squeaky door open slowly, and said, "Gerald, my name is Joseph Wellington. I'm the new administrator here. I hear you have some concerns you'd like to address with me." A smell of body odor smacked me in the face and I immediately considered vomiting.

Gerald was sitting in a wheelchair in the dark room. His television was loud and I wondered if he heard me. "Gerald, my name is Joseph Wellington and….." he interrupted me, "Yeah, yeah, I heard you." When I got close enough to him, I noticed that he had below knee amputations to both of his legs. He had a ratty beard, long greasy hair, and rough skin that wrinkled around his eyes. Gerald was forty-two years old but his rough life of additions and homelessness gave him the appearance of a gentleman of advanced years.

"What can I do for you sir," I proceeded.

"You know that maintenance man you have here? He walked into my room, threatened to 'kick my ass', and told me that he was going to make sure that I didn't get my medicine."

"How did a conversation like that get started?"

"Why does it matter? The last time he hit me that bitch over your nurses told me that I should stay out of his way."

"Gerald, I'm terribly sorry. That is not how I permit business to be conducted. Would you please tell me what happened the last time and this time in as much detail as you can possibly remember."

"Don't talk to me like a fucking 100 year old. My memory isn't my problem," he said while turning to the nurse, "Get me my damned methadone. I know it is five minutes late."   "I'll be right back," she said as she rushed out of the room.

"Gerald," I said pulling out a pen to write on my notepad, "can you tell me what happened last time? I need to know specific details including who you told and how they responded."

Gerald proceeded to tell me the details about how the maintenance man struck him in the face with an open hand after he called the maintenance man an idiot. The maintenance man, allegedly, didn't like being told that the residents were not happy with his performance. Gerald claimed that he told LaToya and she blamed the incident on him, personally, and told him to stay out of the maintenance man's way next time.

This time, however, he alleged that the maintenance man threatened to beat him up really bad and blame it on his roommate. Gerald was frightened. He admitted, "When my methadone wears off, I have a hard time seeing straight. I get angry, cranky, nervous, and frightened very easily. If I had my medicine I wouldn't even care but he threatened me with my medicine."

The nurse walked in and handed Gerald his methadone with a glass of water. He swallowed the methadone without the water and then told me to give him a minute before he continued the conversation.

"Gerald, we do not tolerate that type of behavior here in this facility. I'm going to do the following: I'm going to suspend the maintenance man while we conduct an investigation and then terminate him if the investigation shows that he poses a risk here. This is our policy."

"Oh, jeez, fella, I don't want to see anyone lose their job. I was a working man myself." His behavior had completely been altered within the matter of a minute. I was puzzled. I wasn't aware that methadone 'kicked in' so fast. Perhaps it was a 'placebo effect' but, either way, his behavior changed dramatically over the course of a full ten minute conversation.

"Gerald, we'll be in touch soon. If you need anything from me, please let the nurses know to call my office and I'll be up to speak with you." I was desperate to leave the room and worried that my clothing had absorbed the smell of his room.

He resumed watching television and reminded me, "Don't forget to close the door when you leave. I can't stand all the crazies staring into my room."

I exited his room into a hallway with lights still flickering. "See, I told you he can be a little rough to deal with. I'll write the statement and get it to you by the end of my shift," Lois said as she proceeded towards the nursing station. I immediately went to the 'clean utility' room and washed my hands. After drying them, I was so thankful to have been out of that room.

Then, I pulled out the Blackberry from the holster on my hip and emailed Shmuey:

> *Before you terminate LaToya, I need her to write a statement regarding the allegation Gerald made against the maintenance man. She'll know what I'm talking about. And, please let her know that it would be in her best interest to have that statement to me by the end of the day. Thank you.*

I returned the phone to the holster and walked to the elevator. I pushed the button and then walked away. The man painting the hallway was still painting in the exact same area. I walked over to him, "You there. My name is Joseph Wellington and I'm the new administrator. Can you tell me who is responsible for fixing all of these flickering light bulbs?"

"That would be Tom and he just left for a family situation."

"Okay, do you know how to change these light bulbs?"

"Yeah, I have changed them before. What? You want me to stop painting and change the light bulbs?"

"That is exactly what I want you to do. Please take care of this immediately. There is no reason why our residents should have to struggle seeing down the hall. What is your name?"

"Manuel."

"Thank you, Manual. I'll be back up here this afternoon to review the lighting situation." He put his head down and nodded in frustration. Then, he stomped away toward the dining room. The painting supplies were left in the middle of the hallway and I stopped him. "Manuel, you can't leave painting supplies out unattended. Please clean these up first and then change the bulbs. When Tom gets back, please have him come to my office."

I proceeded towards the elevator and pushed the button. It was breakfast time. Yet, the dining rooms were empty. There were two staff members on the entire floor and one of them worked in maintenance. I decided to tell the new director of nursing when she arrived of this concern. My plate was getting more full by the minute.

The elevator took me downstairs and opened to a busy floor. The staff members were busy, the residents were up and moving about, and I saw two department managers walking around. They smiled at me and I smiled back.

On the way past LaToya's office, I noticed that the light was on and the door opened. There was a thin woman sitting at the desk with long black hair. She looked up at me and said, "You must be Dr. Wellington. I'm Chris your new DON. Not to worry, I was the DON here many years ago and have served as the DON for another facility in JAR's portfolio."

"It is a pleasure to meet you. The corporate office has briefed you of the problems we face here at this facility?" I asked in a very direct tone.

"Yes, they have. I have everything under control, Dr. Wellington. Latisha Howard will be here shortly and we'll get this place running on the straight and narrow." She brimmed with confidence and excitement. Then she emptied a briefcase of notepads and pens onto her new desk. "I'm going to let you get settled in and then we'll meet at some point after the morning meeting."

"The meeting is in two minutes right?"

I looked down at my watch and it was two minutes from 9am. "You are absolutely right," I said as I walked very fast to the office and picked up speed to the conference room afterwards. It was 9:01am when I arrived.

"Dr. Wellington, it would appear that you are late," said Latrice in a joking tone. "You guys got me." The room was quiet. Chris entered the room wearing dress clothing attire and a white half-lab coat.

"Team, before we get started, I would like to announce that LaToya is no longer with us. The new….." I stopped mid-sentence when the room became engorged with clapping from the team. "Okay. Now, now. I want to introduce your new Director of Nursing, Chris."

"Hi guys," she said with familiarity.

"Chris, you should never have left us. Things have gone downhill fast," LaShawna said. Everyone in the room knew Chris from before and there was a small reunion discussion.

Chris then intervened, "Okay, team, we have a lot of work we have to do in a very short amount of time. I'm going to need everyone here a minimum of twelve hours per day six days per week for three weeks. Are you with me on this?"

Everyone agreed, except Latrice. "Chris, I don't have babysitting past 6 and the weekends will be really hard unless I can bring him to work with me."

"Done. Feel free to bring him to work and we'll have the receptionist plan 'day care' in the evenings and on the weekends," Chris interrupted her. My comfort level was growing with Chris in the building.

We discussed the current resident census, maintenance issues, and then I let Chris take over the meeting. She was a master at this. She moved quickly and had a solid command of the room. And, she didn't have to bully anyone to get it done. I don't impress easily and she definitely impressed me.

Later that morning, Latisha Howard, the corporate regional nurse arrived. She was a short, unimpressive, black woman wearing clothing too large for her bigger frame. Her hair was short and she wore large rimmed glasses.

When she got settled in to one of the chairs at the conference table in my office, she pulled her high heel shoes off and remained barefoot. He shoes were far too small for her feet.

"So, Dr. Wellington, I received a telephone call from you yesterday and didn't have a chance to respond. I'm sorry. What's going on?"

"Yesterday's telephone call was urgent, Latisha. I have addressed the issue and will take it from here. Meanwhile, I am very pleased with Chris. She is real go-getter and has a real command of the team already. I'm going to stay as far out of the way as possible while keeping a close tab on progress. If you need anything from me, please let me know."

"We knew you'd love Chris. A lot of people have personality conflicts with LaToya so that wasn't a surprise there. Chris'll do a great job!"

"Wait a minute. Are you saying that the corporate office believes I wanted LaToya out of this facility because of a personality conflict?"

"Shmuey wanted to make sure that he protected both of you because he said he has a lot of respect for both of you. There's nothing wrong with being a little headstrong and both of you are headstrong."

"I hate to break it to you Latisha, but I wanted her gone because of the mess we're in at this facility."

"Okay, Dr. Wellington, you seem really upset. Why don't we resume this later today, okay?"

"Yes, I am getting more and more upset that this DON was never flagged as problem. We can resume this later. I need to see the last six months of your corporate consultant reports by the end of today. Will that be a problem?"

She reached down for her bag, pulled out her laptop and asked if the email address to the administrator's computer was the same. I gave it to her, anyway. She set the laptop on the desk and started typing. "They're going to come in several emails so that it doesn't flag as 'spam'. Let me know if you miss some of them."

I turned to the computer on my right and opened the Outlook Express. Her emails popped up right away. Then, I highlighted them and hit 'forward' and sent them to my private email address. I would need to review these later to determine how the corporate office missed all of the problems at this building. *Chris can scrub the building clean now and I can prevent this from happening again if I find out where the problems are and get them fixed*, I thought to myself.

"I'm going to Chris' office now if you need me for anything. Let me know if you have questions about the reports. Most administrators need my help with the clinical terms," she said.

"Not to worry, Latisha, I have a PhD in Pharmacology. I'm sure I can manage." She smiled and said, "I'm sure you can." Then she leaned over, picked her shoes up from the floor and walked barefoot out of the office, exposing her swollen ankles.

I turned back to the computer and scrolled through the emails. There was an email from Sarah Dustfy:

Hi Dr. Wellington. I apologize for not getting back to you right away. I spoke with Shmuey and he told me about the personality conflict between LaToya and you. Therefore, we are reassigning her to one of our smaller facilities and returning the DON that was at that facility before her. We know that the two of you will get along. She is all business, too. Let me know if there is anything else I can do for you.

I stared at the computer screen. My heart raced and pounded in my chest. My eyes drooped and I pushed my head backwards, closed my eyes, and took a deep breath. Then I squeezed both of my hands as tight as I could. I envisioned Pug Puppies running in a field and playing with a group of Piglets in medium size grass, a bright sun, plenty of wind, and a cool clear serene stream flowing just within the distance.

As I moved my head back to the normal position, I was relaxed and closed the email opting to not respond until I had time to compose myself thoroughly.

After lunch, a small bowl of soup that was procured from the kitchen, a tall thin woman with long blond hair walked into my office without knocking. She looked like a Swedish model. "Hi, I'm Sally from xxxxxxxx Hospice. We have 36 of your residents on hospice and we like to keep a close relationship with the administrators of the nursing homes we work with. Do you have a minute?"

"Hi, I'm Dr. Wellington. Did you say you have 36 patients on hospice here?"

"Yes. That may seem like a lot but you have a large census."

"That is a lot. Wow. Do you have a card?"

"Sure, let me get you one," she said as she reached into her Coach briefcase, "We also like to remind new administrators that the owner of our hospice is a best friend of Joseph Rackman. JAR Management doesn't permit usage of any other hospice so you can find us pretty easily when a referral needs to be made if you ever lose my card." She handed me the glossy card with her newly manicured hands, displaying a large square cut diamond ring on her wedding finger.

"Okay. Do you know if the residents are asked what hospice they would prefer to use?" Her smile now turned to a frown of suspicion. I had obviously crossed the line with my questions. "That shouldn't be an issue. As I understand it, Mr. Rackman only permits privileges to our hospice company."

"Not a problem. I was just checking." She leaned over my desk, exposing her large bosom, and said, "I hope this isn't out of line but if you ever want to grab a drink sometime, let me know. My cell phone is on the back of the card."

"Thanks Sally. I might take you up on that." She turned around and walked out of the office slowly.

"Whoa! Careful with that one, Dr. Wellington," Jane said as she walked into the office, "I ran to Wendys and got you a better lunch than that kitchen gave you. You do like the Double Stack right?" She was right. I did like the double stack from Wendys. And, frankly, it tasted a hell of a lot better than the soup I just ate.

"I have only been here a week and you know me like a book," I said. "Hey, I was going there anyways and saw that crummy soup on your desk. You eat up. You have made a lot of progress here so far. We need you healthy."

Jane still had her snow boots on. They were black with a little fur at the top. I had never seen her without high heels. She and my wife had now been talking daily and I could tell she was comfortable with me. "Let me get out of these boots and I'll be right back in to give you the skinny on Ms. Loosepants there." She was referring to Sally, the hospice representative.

When she returned, with her trademark red high heels, she sat down at a chair across from the desk and began to tell a story. "When this facility was bought by JAR Management, we had four hospice companies that were here pretty regularly. We never had more than five or six hospice patients at any given time. Then, LaToya was brought into the facility a week after the purchase. JAR Management cancelled privileges for all hospice companies and brought in a new hospice company. My daughter is a nurse for one of the hospice companies. She tells me that xxxxxxxx Hospice is taking on patients without them really qualifying and then falsifying documentation to boost payments for patients that never qualified to begin with. Most of their patients never die within the six months of reimbursement. LaToya squashed all resistance by the other staff."

"Are you telling me that this hospice company is fraudulent?"

"I'm saying that something is fishy. But, that is not where it ends Dr. Wellington. Two months ago, one administrator got curious and started asking questions and they fired him. Now, I overheard you asking questions and Ms. Loosepants decided to put the moves on you like she did to him. Take my advice here, lead her on, don't ask questions, and never take her up on any offers."

"This is so much to take in. Jane, thank you for keeping me in the loop. Your information and communication is more valuable than you could possibly know," I said. My headache returned. It was obvious to me that my blood pressure prescription was not working and I would need to visit my physician. *As soon as she leaves I'll take my blood pressure*, I thought to myself.

"By the way, your wife said we need to double date. You need to meet my Roger." She winked, "And, you'll love Roger."

"Anytime. Let's finish the survey so I have more free time on my hands and then we'll go. Our treat." She smiled and reminded me to stay out of the way of the hospice company. Then, she headed towards her office.

When she closed the door behind her, I pulled out my automatic blood pressure wrist cuff and sat back. I pushed the start button and relaxed. The device beeped. The readings were not a shock to me – 160/102. I released the cuff and returned it to the inside flap of my briefcase.

Meanwhile, I reread the 'reportable' forms I write this morning for LaToya. Then, I remembered that I had not received the copied file from Sharice. I placed the 'reportable' in my briefcase and decided to send it to the state, as of yet.

"Jane," I said on the intercom, "Would you please call Sharice and ask her where the file I requested is?"

"Right away sir," her usual response filled the telephone intercom.

Moments later, Sharice walked in with a large brown expanding folder. "Here at the documents, Dr. Wellington. If there is anything else you need, please let me know. Can I take this file to my office now?"

"Of course. I'm heading out for the night shortly. You have a great night."

"Does that mean we don't have to stay later this evening?"

"Well, Sharice, that depends. Do you have unfinished work that has to get done?"

"Dr. Wellington, if that is the standard by which you measure, then we'll never leave this facility. There is always work that is left undone."

"I see. You are right about that. You can head home at the usual time, then. Thanks, again, for the file," I smiled at her. She smiled back with her bright white teeth showing. Sharice was different from the rest of the team. There was no doubt about that.

Note: The hospice company that is mentioned here actually was charged with fraud and the CEO of that company has been incarcerated for defrauding the Medicare system. Several of the staff members of that agency, including "Sally", were convicted, as well, for fraud and conspiracy. The last time I had any communication with that agency was with the owner, then indicted, and he indicated that he was selling the agency. I have no further follow-up.

Day 5

"Good morning, Dr. Wellington," said Chris when I walked through the door. "Holy begeezis, you scared the hell out of me," I said in a stern tone.

"I tend to do that, Dr. Wellington. My voice can be a little loud."

"Why the hell are you waiting at my office door at 5:30am?" I said and then backed off. "Wait a minute, I meant to say, 'Thank god someone is here waiting at my door at this time and actually working'." Her scowl turned to a smile.

"Apparently, Latisha didn't tell you about me. I will be here 18 hours each day until this building clears. I don't sleep much and have never needed much sleep," she said. Her large brown eyes and perky face certainly justified what she said. Even at this hour, she looked proper with dress clothing and a half lab white coat.

"I see you are a Starbucks gal," I noted as I pointed to her Venti cup of coffee, noting that she was not wearing any jewelry. "What's your pleasure?"

"Oh, give me a Caramel Macchiato any day and I'm happy," and with that we walked into my office. She had several notepads with her and a stack of manila folders.

I put my coffee down and she saw the writing on the glass. "Oh, so you are a Macchiato fan, too. Good man."

"Before we get started, how did you know that I would be here at 5:30am?" I had never arrived that early at any facility before and I certainly hadn't told anyone in the building that I would be here. "Oh, I wasn't waiting here for you. I was trying to get into the copy room and you just happened to pop up."

I glared at her with suspicion. After all, I gave her a set of keys to the entire property. She had access to everything. "Let me be fair in telling you that I find that a little hard to believe. You have a set of keys to the entire property."

She smiled with a playful deviousness. "You got me. I saw you coming into the building and decided to wait for you and greet you. I do need to talk to you, though." She laid all of her items on the conference table and walked over to the desk where she sat in a guest chair.

I worried and then remember that I brought a bottle of Xanax with me in case the day got out of hand. My mind stopped racing as soon as I remembered that the bottle was in my briefcase. I pulled the rolling desk chair back and sat down. "What's on your mind, kiddo?" It felt as if we were already at the point in our relationship where we could be playful.

"You need to promise me that what I tell you is completely confidential," she now looked concerned.

"Are you planning on killing yourself or someone else?" I asked in all seriousness. I had seen suicides amongst staff. Her look in reply told me she as unsure as to why the question was even asked. "Of course, I will keep your confidence. As long as my trust is not betrayed, you have my word."

"Latisha thinks you are here to get her fired. She wants me to dig up as much dirt on your as possible so that you'll get tossed first."

"Wait a minute, you're telling me," I said before she interrupted me. "There's more, Dr. Wellington. I was told by Shmuey to watch you closely, too. They only do that when they want to fire someone."

I looked her, squinted my eyes a little bit, and then took a deep breath. She looked back and her eyes watered. It was obvious to me that she was worried I would breach her confidence and get her in trouble. "Give me one moment," and I stood up and walked the length of the office to close the door.

When I returned to the desk, I sat in the guest chair next to her. "Can you and I talk for a moment and can I guarantee that I have your complete confidence?"

"Dr. Wellington, you need to know something. I would never breach your confidence. I'm telling you what is happening because – well – um, because," she looked worried again. "Promise me that won't tell her that I told you anything?"

"Chris, sweetie, we are starting to circle the airport here. You have my word."

"Jane really likes you a lot and she is one of my best friends. She told me that she is confident that out of all of the administrators this facility has had, you are by far the best and she doesn't want to lose you."

"That is really sweet. And, I have to tell you that if Jane and you are friends than you are a new friend. I don't know why this place is like a minefield but, for whatever reason, it just is. If you wouldn't mind telling them that you have found nothing, I'd completely appreciate that."

"Oh, you have my word on that. They're getting nothing negative out of me. But, you should know that this means when the survey closes they will attempt to fire me. Will you protect me from that?" She was intensely serious here. This meeting was more of a quid pro quo than a 'heads up'. I gave her my word that I would protect her from termination with all the authority that I was provided.

"Chris, I would like to also tell you that I'm not worried about being terminated here. You will be the only one that knows this but I am working on retainer with a contract that indicates a termination, with or without cause, will result in the company forfeiture of their retainer," and I watched her smile when she heard this.

"Jane's right. You are a smart cookie!"

And, with that statement, she stood up and collected her belongings and marched out of the office. Although she didn't ask, she closed the door behind her and kept moving. I quickly reached into my briefcase and wrote in the leather-bound executive journal, '*Chris came to me today and notified me of the situation with the corporate office. The regional nurse wants me gone and fears for her own job because of how poorly she has done here and the regional operations manager wants to find any dirt on me. This place is a warzone. I will need to meet with the owner in the very near future – face to face – to let him know what my findings are and how we need to proceed organizationally to prevent this from happening in the future. Meanwhile, I'm confident Chris can get this facility's clinical deficiencies cleared with integrity'.*

I returned the journal to my briefcase and pulled out a notepad. The notepad was covered in scribbled and barely legible, even to me, notes from last night.

Last night, I pored over all of the consultant reports from the regional nurse. Since Latisha didn't alter any of these documents, as she sent them while sitting in front of me, I wasn't shocked with the horrors I saw.

On one report, she wrote: *'Resident death occurred as a direct result of infected wounds that she acquired in the facility. As I understand it, the family is not involved. I made the changes in the EMR (electronic medical record) to reflect the wounds acquired in the hospital instead. I don't see any litigation or risk here.'*

On another report, she wrote: *'The DON (director of nursing) took care of the nosey restorative coordinator. She brought in her own person and now we can make sure the documentation reflects the actual orders. All documentation prior to this has been fixed. We should make sure that HR (human resources) is aware of this to avoid risk.'*

There were pages and pages of these statements, all marked 'Confidential, Attorney-Client Privileged Information'. I knew I would need to meet with Joseph Rackman. The owners of the facilities rarely get so involved that they read the nurse consultants' reports. It was my intention to show him that this facility grew more tiresome in the efforts to provide good care, while being profitable, because of the failed efforts of the consultant.

The computer was turned off last night and I had to wait for it to boot up. Once the email application was opened, I began typing:

Dear Mr. Rackman:

Good morning to you sir. I need to speak with you about this facility. We now have a DON in place that I believe can manage the clinical issues of the past. I

will maintain a working plan of action file to ensure that we remain on targeted
schedule for compliance and avoid decertification.

That being said, we need to set up a meeting to discuss your regional team. I am
quite worried that this team is.....

I stopped typing and hit the 'backspace' button. I then held it down and erased the entire email. *He would have to know about these documents, especially with the amount of litigation this facility is facing*, I thought to myself. My right leg bounced with nervousness and anxiety and I reached into the briefcase and pulled out the bottle of Xanax. I put one of them in my mouth and downed it with the coffee.

I proceeded with:

Dear Mr. Rackman:

When you receive this email, please give me a call. There are some serious things we need to discuss. Thanks.

Kind Regards,

Dr. W.

I hit the 'send' button and stood up. I would need to discuss these things in person and not via an email. Since I came in early to see how the facility operated overnight and to finish paperwork, I started my rounds onto the floors.

There were very few staff members and the stench was unbearable. *Today, I will tackle this staffing problem*, I made a mental note.

When I returned to the office, I opened my email application to see that Joseph had responded, '*Let's talk at 10am. Call me at the office.*' I penciled his name into my open planner for 10am and also keyed the meeting into my Blackberry so that a 'reminder' buzz would go off five minutes before the meeting was to begin.

I glanced back at the 'At-A-Glance' planner that remained open on my desk. In almost every corner of the open pages writing was scribbled. There were 'to do lists' and 'meetings' and 'reminders'. I reached for my yellow highlighter and scrawled across both pages, '*Overwhelmed*'. Then, I felt the nervousness subside.

"Dr. Wellington," Mary said after knocking on the door as softly as she could, "Why are you here so early?" I looked at her and said, "I might ask the same of you."

"To be honest, you bugged me yesterday so I wasn't able to get all of my work done. I decided I was going to beat you here in case you interrupted me again," and then she laughed. "No, I'm just teasing. I couldn't sleep so I decided to come to the office."

"I'm glad you are here, Mary. I have some questions for you. Please take a seat," I responded as she walked to the conference table.

Mary wore a black blouse with cat hair showing. She smelled of cigarette smoke. And, she carried her trademark coffee mug that said, '*I should be in Florida with a rich man*'. She pulled the chair from the conference table, set her coffee mug down, and then took a seat.

I grabbed a notepad, both personnel files on my desk, and walked over to the conference table. "Here are your files back," I said as I handed them over to her. Then, I sat down, "but I need to ask you some questions about them."

"I knew this was coming," she responded nervously. "Dr. Wellington, I told them not to strip these files. I said that we would get in trouble with the state because everything was missing." She kept going and going without my first question ever being asked.

"Mary, slow down. Are you telling me that someone told you to strip these files of all pertinent information?"

"Shmuey came in here yesterday morning and told me to take out all information other than the basics for all managers. He also wanted me to give him LaToya's entire file. When I refused, he said he wanted to see it. He even removed her application for employment and left her resume. I'm supposed to let him know if you ask for any personnel files."

"Mary, I like you. If you value your employment here, and your freedom from incarceration, I'm going to recommend that you not follow his advice going forward.

You need to return all documents to these files and do not tell him that I requested personnel files. Can I trust that you on that?"

"What if he?" I interrupted her, "Can I trust you, Mary?"

"You can trust me. I won't say anything," she responded. "Great," I said, "and now I need payroll records for LaToya."

"Dr. Wellington, we don't keep records the way you think. Well, we do, but not for LaToya. She has a special arrangement."

"What kind of special arrangement?"

"LaToya has a $135,000 base salary and then she is given $65 per hour for each hour she spends working on the clinical floor when there are staffing challenges."

"Unbelievable! That is why this facility has very little staff. She was working the floors and collecting a massive paycheck," I retorted.

"Shmuey instructed me to not hire any additional staff members and that LaToya would work the floor. But, can you keep a secret?"

"Sure. We've already come this far," I responded with sarcasm.

"LaToya was never here when she documented that she worked the floor." I lowered my eyebrows questioning that statement. "If you don't believe me, check for any documentation with her signature anywhere by comparing the 'extra payments' in the payroll records. The administrator doesn't sign off on payroll for LaToya. Shmuey does."

"Mary, you are a treasure trove of information. Look, this conversation never happened. Agreed?" I nodded my head up and down seeking agreement.

"For sure, Dr. Wellington. For sure." She stood up, picked up her coffee, and proceeded out of the door, "Would you pull the door shut behind you Mary? Thanks!"

The door shut and my pen moved at lightning speed across the notepad. Then, another knock came at the door, "Dr. Wellington," the muffled sound said, "May I come in?" This was not a face I recognized.

I waved my hand with permission to enter. "Hello, Dr. Wellington. We haven't met. I'm Cassandra the marketing director here," she said. Cassandra stood at 5'9, had long blown out straight black hair, work a black dress that clung to her caramel colored skin, and wore a necklace that draped into her bosom beneath her dress.

"Hi Cassandra, it's nice to meet you. I haven't seen you here at all. Were you on vacation?"

"No. I've been at the local hospitals marketing our facility. It's tough out there right now. Everyone is pushing for the same patients. Which brings me to why I'm here. I need to get into the safe underneath your desk. Did Shmuey give you the code yet?"

"I have the code. You don't have a company credit card for marketing events?"

"No, I have a company credit card. There is, off the record, a social worker at xxxxxx hospital that we pay to get us the Medicare residents. Without him, I'm not sure what we would do with our reputation," she said with a sad tone.

"We are paying the social workers for admissions?"

"Um, yeah. Is that a problem, sir?" she now sounded sarcastic. "Well, Cassandra, that is a problem. It's illegal."

"I'll just call Shmuey to get the money. This is ridiculous. I shouldn't have to come in here and explain why I need every dime," she now got angrier. "Actually, Cassandra, you do have to explain why you need every dime of a company's money."

Cassandra turned around and stormed out of my office, slamming my door behind her. The glass in the door rattled. The sound of the slamming door was loud. Under normal circumstances, I would have followed her. In this case, it had already become clear to me that I was not in charge of this facility. I was merely paid to be the face of the facility until they could pay off the surveyors that had 'requested my services'.

I looked back down at the notepad and continued scrawling my notes. This time, I wrote, '*Need to keep a close tab on payment for admissions. This is very strange. Cassandra unhappy that she was denied funds to pay off a social worker and slammed door hard*'. It was getting close to the meeting time and I needed to prepare.

After the meeting, one in which Chris ran with the expertise and precision of a specialist, I returned to the administrative offices area. Jane was sitting at her desk and looked up, phone on her ear, smiled and waved while mouthing 'good morning'.

I mouthed 'good morning' back to her and walked into the office. After I sat down at the desk, I heard a knock on the door and Jane was standing in the doorframe. "Good morning Jane. Come on in," I said with excitement. "Good morning, Dr. Wellington. How are you today?"

"The day started off very fast today, Jane. How are you?"

"I'm doing well. The phone is ringing non-stop today. Anyway, Joseph Rackman called for you and said he would like for you to call him. He sounded angry," she said as she nodded her head.

"This sounds like a common theme with this company," I said laughing. "But, even so, I wasn't supposed to call him until 10am. Maybe he forgot to reread his own email to me. Let me give him a call."

"Very good sir. Let me know if you need anything," as she walked out of the office and closed the door silently.

I pulled the telephone closer to me, looked up Joseph's number on my Blackberry, and dialed the office phone. A mouse-like voice answered the phone, "Mr. Rackman's office."

"Good morning. This is Dr. Wellington returning Joseph Rackman's telephone call," I said as professional as possible.

"Yes sir. He is waiting for you. I'll transfer you in now."

The phone rang twice and Joseph picked up with a deep voice. His voice was scratchy and he sounded as if he just rolled out of bed. "Joseph, what is all this business about you making changes without checking with me?"

"Okay, Mr. Rackman, we're going to start out by taking it down a notch. I don't know what you are talking about," I said nervously.

"My friend Sally called and told me that you're planning on changing the hospice services. Are you out of your fucking mind?"

"I'm not sure I understand what you are talking about," I responded with all sincerity.

"For every hospice patient, we get a small percentage as a friendly referral bonus. You, if you stay, get a percentage of that referral bonus. You got it? Understand? For god sakes, you have a fucking doctorate, this shouldn't be fucking rocket science to you."

"I think that is the least of my concerns right now. Can we talk about this facility and the concern over it getting decertified before we start jumping to conclusions about what I have or have not said?" my voice grew deeper with frustration.

"Go ahead. What do you want?" he sounded annoyed.

"First and foremost, I have a problem with the regional director of operations here. He has sex with the director of nursing on her desk and when he is caught, he screams at me. Then, he tells all of the staff her to keep a close eye on me. How in the world am I to conduct business in a position of authority with that happening?" he attempted to interrupt me and I proceeded. "Then, the nurse consultant reports for the past six months have noted that she is fraudulently documenting and altering records. There is nothing in these reports of planning and real long term solutions. The facility has made sweetheart deals with the director of nursing to the point that it has nearly bankrupted the building's NOI each month. Did you know that she has made, in six months, a total of $110,000? Were you aware that she forced a resident to leave without paperwork and now we are at risk for litigation? Are you aware of the amount of litigation that is in this facility because of the incompetence of the regional staff members and poor selection and management of department managers in the facility?"

"You sound like you have a problem with the way I run my business," he responded in an attempt to intimidate.

"I absolutely have a problem with the way you are running this facility. The residents are receiving poor care because your regional operations manager told the HR manager her to stop hiring staff so the DON that he was having an affair with could work shifts 'on paper I might add' and get paid additional dollars? He's been using this place as his personal piggybank to pay people for sex. I absolutely have a problem with the fact that you asked me to fix this nursing home and I have no authority to do so. We have a problem here. No, let me correct this Joseph, you have a problem," I said as I wrote in my notepad a reminder that if I was terminated I would owe nothing in the initial retainer payments to the company. That calmed my nerves.

"Be at my office this afternoon," he said gruffly and hung up.

I called his office back and the mouse-like voice picked up once again. "I need to speak with Joseph. I believe we were disconnected." She placed me on hold and a moment of silence later returned, "Mr. Rackman states he would like to see you this afternoon."

"Please communicate with Mr. Rackman that I will not be coming to his office. I have a lot of work to do. If he wishes to meet with me in person, I am at the facility and he can reach me there."

She said, "Please hold a moment and let me check his calendar."

"No. Let him know that I said that and if he has a problem with that, he can call me tomorrow to work out a date and time that works for my schedule."

"Please hold."

A very angry Mr. Rackman took the call, "You son of a bitch. Shmuey is my nephew and if you think for one minute that I'm going to fire him you're out of your fucking mind. As for the regional nurse, we can talk about her this afternoon at my office."

"There is nothing to talk about. I want a decision made and I'm not coming to your office so that we can pretend that I'm intimidated by you. Make a decision here. This facility can't wait. You can decide to toss her and bring someone aboard that can work with integrity or you can keep her and shutter the facility doors and face bankruptcy – and your name splashed across page one of the newspaper."

"I'll call you back," he responded and hung up the phone. I looked back down at the notepad where I reminded myself of the contract retainer fee being forfeited in case of a termination. I felt calm. But, apparently, that is not how it appeared through the window.

"Are you okay?" Jane said with her voice muffled behind the glass window of the door. I simply nodded yes. She smiled and walked away from the door. I pulled a tissue out of the tissue box and blew my nose while audibly saying, "I gotta give up caramel. It's just making the sinuses worse."

Then, I pulled my scarf off of the coat hanger and draped it around my neck and down my shoulders. I turned to the computer and opened up the email application. In front of me sat an email from Shmuey, '*We need to talk*'. I resolved that I would not call him and I would not respond to this email. He would need to seek me out in order.

A knock at the door came from Jane, "Dr. Wellington, Shmuey is on the phone and he is not happy. He asked for 'Dr. Jackass' in reference to you." Then, she chuckled, "Boy you really got under his skin fast. Don't do anything to get yourself fired, okay?"

I smiled and picked up the phone, "This is Dr. Wellington. How may I help you?"

"Give the code to the safe to the marketing director when she comes back to your office," Shmuey said.

"Absolutely not. There is over $20,000 in that safe and I'm not going to give the code to someone not responsible for the security of such dollars."

"Why are you being such an asshole? She needs the money to land an admission and she told you that."

"And, I told her what I'm going to tell you – you cannot do that it is illegal. Period."

"Fine, I'll be there in an hour. When she comes back to the office, tell her I'm stuck in traffic but I'll be there shortly," he said with a chillingly calm voice.

"I'll tell her that but I'm telling you right now that I want no part of this 'deal' that you are striking. It can land a lot of people in the slammer and you should know that."

Shmuey wasn't interested in hearing the entire statement because he hung up right after I said 'telling you'. I finished the line to reassure myself that I would have no part of this. Then, I returned to the email application and hit 'respond' and wrote:

I still need the statement from LaToya as quickly as possibly regarding the Gerald incident.

Then, I hit 'send' and stood up. I needed to get some fresh air. "Jane, I'm heading to Starbucks. Do you want anything?"

"Oh, it's that kind of morning. Can you get me a Passion Iced Tea, sweetened?" she said. "You bet. I'll be back in twenty minutes."

The outside air felt so good. The heavy cold entering my lungs lowered my climbing body temperature that rose with each frustrating conversation.

When I returned to the facility, Jane smiled at me and said, "Get enough fresh air for the both of us?" I laughed, handed her the drink, and walked to the office. My office light was off, as if I had left for the day. I turned the light back on and wondered if I had turned it off when I left.

"Dr. Wellington, I hope you don't mind. I turned off your light when you left. You seemed frustrated and I didn't want anyone wasting their time paging you," said Chris as she followed me into the office. "We have a problem. Gerald on Unit 2 is claiming that the maintenance man hit him."

"Did he say when the event happened?"

"Yes. He said the maintenance man, Tom, came to his room and struck him in the chest this morning."

"Chris, that's not possible. I suspended the maintenance man yesterday. He hasn't been back to the facility," I said with confidence.

"Oh, I wonder if that is public knowledge. He came in this morning and said he spoke with the corporate office and they told him to return to the facility," she said in frustration. "This is what this company does all the time, Dr. Wellington. They override my decisions a lot, too."

I looked down at the desk and wrote, 'Call Sarah Dustfy about Tom's suspension being lifted without my consent'. Then, I told Chris I appreciated her letting me know and that she would need to write a statement. "Not to worry, I have already opened an investigation file."

"Fantastic! Thanks, Chris!"

I grabbed my Blackberry from my belt holster and searched for Sarah Dustfy's direct telephone line. I hit the 'call' button and listened to the ringing.

"Sarah Dustfy here," said the chipper voice on the other end of the line.

"Hi Sarah. This is Dr. Wellington. I received word today that a man I suspended, Tom in maintenance, was notified by the corporate office he was allowed to return and should report back to work today. Please tell me that this isn't true."

"Dr. Wellington, it is absolutely true. You had no right to suspend him without getting approval from the regional operations manager."

"Are you telling me that I have been placed here, as a licensed professional, to receive marching orders? That won't work Sarah. As far as I'm concerned that is a breach of contract."

"It isn't a breach of contract. We told you in the beginning that you cannot make any disciplinary actions without checking with us first."

"Sarah, I'm walking to that man's maintenance office in two minutes to tell him he is suspended. If I hear that you are forcing me to bring him back again, I'll file a complaint with the state personally and call this a breach."

"Let me call Shmuey before you do anything else. We don't want to create conflict here," she said with a voice of desperation and a placating tone at the same time.

"I'm doing it with or without Shmuey's permission. Sarah, there is a reason that nursing home administrators are required to be licensed. This is one of those times that the requirement has a proven reason to be in place. Shame on this company for making a decision like reversing a suspension of a man who abused a resident and shame on you for making that call and justifying it."

I hung up the phone without any further desire to have a conversation about this. I raised myself from the desk, felt dizzy, and sat back down in the chair. Thinking back on the morning, I had consumed nothing to eat. Thankfully, inside my briefcase was a protein bar. I ate this and rested for a fifteen minutes until the dizziness stopped. My undershirt was drenched in sweat. I closed the blinds to the window on the door and removed my undershirt and dressed myself again with the button up shirt.

I rolled the undershirt up and placed it underneath my desk.

Then, I proceeded out of the office. I was stopped abruptly by Cassandra, "I spoke with Shmuey and he said you were to give me the code to the safe." She smiled mischievously. "Dr. Wellington, I'm on a schedule here. Can you speed up?" I laughed at her, inappropriately, "You really think I would give you the code to an executive safe? Shmuey knows better. That being said, he did tell me to let you know that he will be here in an hour or so."

"This is seriously fucked up. If I lose my bonus because of your slow ass, we're going to have a problem."

"No, Cassandra. You're the one with the problem. Now, if you will excuse me, I have something to take care of." I exited the administrative offices while she pulled out her cell phone and dialed.

The hallway was filled with a line of patients outside of one room. The patients all looked like they were waiting outside of a school to enter their classrooms. "Dr. Wellington, the Podiatrist is here. Please ignore the line," said Latrice. "I have to organize this because LaToya fired the nurse that helped the podiatrist out when he came."

"No worries, Latrice," I said. She smiled at me and said, "Things here are going to be okay. At church last night, we prayed for this facility." I smiled at her. "I'm sure they will be, too." Only, inside, I was not sure that things would be okay.

The maintenance office was the second to last door in the hallway. The door was locked. Instead of getting a key, I knocked on the door and Tom, the maintenance man, opened the door. "Yes, what do you want?" he said to me in a very stern tone.

"Tom, while this may be hard for you to believe, you remain suspended until we can complete this investigation. A resident has alleged that you abused him. He has alleged that you abused him again this morning when you were not supposed to be here. I need you to leave this facility immediately," I instructed him.

"I was told I could return to this facility today."

"Tom, I'm not being arbitrary and I'm not being hostile. If you do not leave, I will have you removed by the police. Let's not take it that far, okay?"

Tom looked down, grabbed his cell phone from his pocket, and dialed. "Sarah, this asshole is telling me I have to leave the premises again. I thought you told me that he doesn't have any authority to do this?" He listened to her for a moment, finished the telephone call, grabbed his jacket, and said to me, "This isn't over." Then, I followed him to the front door to ensure that he left the building.

I returned to the main area on the first floor, pushed the call button to the elevator, and looked around. The first floor was much busier than I had seen it since I arrived. I saw nurses moving around quickly and nursing aides appeared busy, as well.

That was completely different when I stepped off of the elevator onto the second floor. The smell was putrid and the residents looked disheveled. Only, today, I noticed

Chris on the second floor directing the nurse on her expectations. "This nursing station needs to remain organized regardless of how busy you think you are. We're going to get you some help here soon," I heard her say from a distance.

"Hi Chris. Would you mind taking a tour with me?" Chris smiled and headed my direction while greeting all of the residents with a 'good morning' and a smile.

"Where would you like to start?" she said. "Let's get started down 2B. I have only been down that hall twice since I have been here. I'm going to get housekeeping actively involved on the second floor while we find staff to actually work it."

"The staffing here is by far the worst part of the problem. Once we have staffing levels normalized, you'll see things change rapidly. No worries. I'm on it." She had just as much energy as she did this morning. The only difference was her hair was scrunched up and behind her head now.

The very first resident room was a gentleman by the name of Omar Guzman. He was a gang member that had a gun shot wound to his back and was considered paralyzed from the waist down. His door was cracked open so we knocked and walked into the room swiftly. Tonya, a nursing assistant covered in tatoos, was on her knees performing oral sex on Mr. Guzman.

Chris and I both apologized and turned around to exit the room when Chris said, "Wait a minute, you're not a visit. What the hell do you think you are doing?"

"Get the fuck out of here and let her finish," said Omar.

Tonya came out a few moments later. "You two didn't see shit. Got that?"

"Um, yes we did young lady," Chris said, "now get your belongings and leave this facility."

"Make me," Tonya said. "Not a problem. Chris pulled out her cell phone and dialed a number. Hello, I have a disgruntled and aggressive employee a xxxxxxxx care center that needs to be removed. Her name?" and she turned to Tonya and said, "What is your name dear?"

"My name is Tonya Martinez," she said sarcastically.

"The young lady says her name is Tonya Martinez. How long will you be? Very well, I'll let her know that you are on your way," and then she turned to Tonya and said,

"Now, we can do this the easy way or the hard way. The police are on their way and you can be physically removed or I can have you walked out on your own terms."

Chris was calm and collected during the entire altercation. "I'll get my shit and go. Am I fired?"

I looked and Chris and Chris looked back at me. "Um, yeah, you are fired. But, you are more than welcome to return as a visitor and cultivate the relationship with this gentleman. But, that won't be today. I wish you well in your future endeavors. You'll get a call from Mary in human resources later today so that you can write a statement or accept the termination without fighting it."

We followed Tonya to employee break room on the second floor where she collected her very large purse and trendy faux fur coat. Sharice watched what happened and offered to walk her out, "I usually get called to walk everyone out when Mary isn't around," she said. Chris and I thanked her.

Chris led me back to Mr. Guzman's room and we knocked. "Mr. Guzman," Chris said, "I know you remember me. I'm the one that fired your last girlfriend for bringing in weed for you."

"Oh, yeah, I know you," he said. "You fire Tonya?"

"Um, she no longer works here. You are welcome to call her if she gave you her number. We also told her that she is welcome to cultivate a relationship with you after today."

"Fuck. You know how long it took me to get that bitch to suck on these nuts? And, that bitch swallows," he said without missing a beat. There was no shame in his voice.

"Okay, well Mr. Guzman, Chris and I have to continue our rounds," I said. I never introduced myself to him and he never asked who I was. Chris looked over at Mr. Guzman and said, "You know, Omar, you don't have to be here if you feel functional. We can help you find a support system in the community so you can live outside of this nursing home."

"Yeah right, words only. Get the fuck out of my room," he said. We both immediately left without responding.

Once outside in the hallway, I asked, "What is his story? He seems so angry."

"I knew Omar as a kid. His parents were good parents. But, he got mixed up with the gangs and then he got shot in a gang shoot out. All of his buddies abandoned him. Now, he gets these young street tough chicks to get close to him and then they do things for him that they shouldn't be doing – illegal drugs, sex, and other stuff," she said as she nodded her head. She looked like a disappointed mother.

We finished the rounds together and then I heard an overhead page, "Dr. Wellington, please report to your office. Dr. Wellington, please report to your office." It was Jane's pleasant and professional voice. I turned to Chris and told her to please have housekeeping take care of the smell on the entire floor and gave her the green light to let Mary in human resources know to start hiring staff right away.

I hopped on the elevator and headed downstairs expecting to find an angry Shmuey in my office. Before I got to the office, Jane signaled to me with a shush finger and waving her arms that he was angry. I raised my hands and put my thumb up for approval. Then, I walked into my office.

"Good morning, Shmuey. How are you today?"

"Don't give me that bullshit. You changed the code on this safe, didn't you," he forcefully asked. "I absolutely changed the code to the safe when I arrived. You wouldn't begrudge me a little protection, would you?" He laughed and snickered, inappropriately, to antagonize him.

He pulled his pants up nervously and rubbed his hand on his nose while I made a mental note to disinfect every inch of the office after he left. "A little protection, eh? You have a wet t-shirt under your desk. It seems to me that you already used protection." He may have intended to frustrate me with his facial expression but, alas, he was not going to get me that easy.

"Shmuey, as much as you would like to think that, we're not the same person. I don't sleep with my team members. That is a rule that every manager should follow. You need to learn that as you grow and develop in your role," I said in a very fatherly tone. He was not grateful for the advice or the 'paternal bullshit' as he called it.

"Open the fucking safe. I'll sign for whatever you need," he said in an attempt to intimidate. "Okay, and you will have to document in the 'reason' section of the form as to why this money was taken. I will need receipts for reconciliation purposes."

"Dr. Wellington, that is not how we do things here. We don't need receipts for 'petty cash' items."

"Normally that is true, but I don't know how much it costs to bribe a hospital discharge planning social worker to screw over a patient and send them to a nursing home against their will." My tone was of condescension and he knew it. He elevated his posture and said, "Now you think you're better than me? You think I wouldn't kick your ass right here in this office?"

"Shmuey, under normal circumstances, I'd say I'd like to see you try. But, you and I both know that in five days I have more information of this facility's illegal activities and that it would be stupid of you to attempt it. You also know that the state has requested me, specifically, so it would be pleasurable for me to pick up the phone and let my friends at the public health department know what happened here."

He looked away from me and at Cassandra, "Let's get out of here Cassandra. We can hit the ATM." Shmuey stormed out of the office in a huff. The body odor seemed to get worse when his arms swung from side to side and the trail of the odor followed him outside of the office.

Once they left, Jane walked into the office spraying room deodorizer, "I'm so proud of you. You have so much integrity. I know why Paula married you." She turned around and walked out of the office.

Later that day, I received a telephone call from Joseph Rackman with two lines, "You can have it your way for now. We'll discuss everything after the building is back in compliance." The phone call was strange because he didn't even know if I was the one on the call. He simply said what he needed to say and hung up.

Unfortunately, I was out of time and had to do a report on the Gerald situation. So, I picked up the telephone and called Mary in human resources directly. She picked up the phone and said, "Mary", as if to identify herself.

"Mary, it's Joseph. I need the personnel file for Tom in maintenance. Would you bring it to me right away and most urgently please," although it sounded like a request, she knew that it was a directive.

"Sure thing, Dr. Wellington. I'll be right there."

Very little time had passed when Mary arrived with file in hand. "As long as we are clear that you don't share with anyone, I'll give you the complete file. I have put all documents in here that belong in here."

"Mary, you and I are developing a great relationship. Please have a seat," I said as she sat down nervously.

"Dr. Wellington, I mean no disrespect. I can't afford to lose my job," as her eyes filled up with tears.

"Mary, I merely want to tell you that you can trust my word. I'm someone that takes my word very seriously and if I tell you that I will keep what you say confidential, you have to trust me. We have to begin with trust here."

Mary leaned over the conference table, half standing from her chair, and reached for the box of tissues. She pulled one out and wiped her eyes. "You don't know what it has been like here. Every single time something goes wrong in this building, the corporate office calls me and threatens me with my job if I don't do exactly what they want."

"I can understand that. If for no other reason than the fact that I'm now here in this building, please double check with me before complying. My professional license is responsible for this facility complying with the regulations and I am not willing to allow that to be compromised. I have to know what is going on in this building to be successful here. Deal?"

"Deal."

"Now, as for Tom's file, I'm going to make sure I get it all back to you in the morning. What time are you leaving for the day?"

"I think I'm going to leave early today."

"Early," I said, "It's already past 5pm." Then we both laughed as she walked out of the room wishing me a good evening.

I reviewed Tom's file and learned that this was not the first time he was accused of abusing a resident. In an effort to not cause any further trouble, I telephone the director of nursing and asked her for the full investigation. "Dr. Wellington, I'll bring it up right away. Between you and I, I think he definitely hit Gerald. Gerald even has bruises to prove it."

"Fair enough. Before we leave, we need to file a formal report with the state and notify the corporate office that we need to issue Tom's termination. We may need to file a police report, as well."

Chris brought the investigation file to my office and I wrote the formal report and faxed it off to the state department of health, personally, to ensure it was actually done.

Intermission

By now, you the reader have probably gotten to understand the frustration that I experienced. This company is not an anomaly, though. The industry standard is to behave in this unethical way. In the 1980s, it was determined by the legislative body in Washington DC that nursing home administrators must be licensed, even as employees, to ensure that companies actually comply with regulations. They underestimated the power of the nursing home owners to leverage 'golden handcuffs' and 'terminations' for non-compliance.

Over the course of the next couple of weeks:

1. I was instructed to hide medical records from a litigant. I ensured that the medical records made it to the litigant.

2. I was instructed to rehire Tom (the maintenance man I ultimately fired for a confirmed abuse situation). The family was never notified by the director of nursing, as her job was threatened, about the situation. In fact, the investigation file disappeared from my desk by the morning when I arrived after submitting the report.

3. I submitted a report to the state with my concerns over the clinical department. While it may seem unprofessional to have done this, it was necessary. I was repeatedly blocked from intervening and making progress in the clinical department by the corporate office. The only way to get this done was by forcing their hands. Not only did I file the report, I then confessed that I was the party that filed it. My report included many issues (not just the death).

4. The falsification of records troubled me so terribly that I ultimately filed complaints against all licensees involved, including the corporate office's intention to cover these up.

5. The company general counsel, after instructing me to break the law repeatedly, had a licensure complaint filed with the state bar by me.

6. The state department of health arrived to the facility to clear deficiencies before a decertification. Shmuey was in the facility, paid the health surveyors, and they cleared the facility of all wrongdoing. This was very close to my 'day 30' that I introduced in the beginning of this book.

7. The hospice company was ultimately brought up on fraud charges and the owner criminally charged. Several of his executive employees were charged, as well. The owner of the nursing home called me, along with all nursing home administrators for his facilities, and instructed us to keep our mouths shut and discharge all residents from this hospice and transition them to another hospice company – "if they still need it" he said.

8. The corporate nurse consultant was ultimately fired after I put up such a complaint about her behavior in the facility. I found her sleeping several times in the second floor office. Later, however, I learned that she was not 'fired' so much as moved to another one of the owner's holdings.

9. I hired many nurses to get the floors completely covered with the appropriate amount of help. The corporation entered the facility and decreased everyone's hours to the lowest possible to avoid having to offer insurance and payments.

10. I fought with the corporate human resources department (Sarah Dustfy) about payroll on many occasions. She instructed Mary to 'trim a little off the top' for everyone's payroll. Thus, if an employee worked 60 hours, Mary would only pay then for 52 to avoid having to pay for more. I filed a complaint with the state wage and hour department.

11. After I discovered the therapy department, in-house, was owned by the nursing home owner, I asked if this was disclosed in the admission agreement. I was told to 'keep my mouth shut' because I was not 'aware of this either'. I never filed a formal complaint but I did instruct the social worker on the premises to let everyone know this when she assisted with signing admission agreements (contracts).

12. After fighting for several weeks with the 'clinical reimbursement coordinator' on forcing therapy services onto residents that couldn't tolerate the amount of services (or equally as horrific, for services that were not required at all), I filed a formal complaint with CMS about the facility's fraudulent billing practices.

13. The corporate office would often call the facility and instruct the social worker to discharge a resident for non-payment and to 'get them out of this building by the end of the day'. I repeatedly intervened and told them that they needed to issue a 30 day notice to the residents. Sadly, I was overridden by the corporation many times by residents being transferred to other facilities against their will or, worse, to homeless shelters.

14. Several of the 'contractors' that serviced the property were owned by the nursing home owner. When I asked if this was disclosed, he became angry with me. I was not so concerned about most of these contracts. The contracts I worried about were the ones that affected the residents – pharmacy, x-ray, medical director, psychiatrist, etc.

Day 29

The day before my departure, I sat in my office working on strategic plans. After all, Shmuey had bribed the public health workers and my focus had now switched to solutions and quality assurance going forward.

"Dr. Wellington, take a look outside. Mr. Rackman is here unannounced," Jane said while standing at my door. My brain scanned every reason why he could possibly be showing up at this facility. He couldn't be here to terminate my contract since I had received the full amount of money per the agreement.

I stood up and walked to front desk, "Mr. Rackman. Good to see you. Come on back."

Joseph walked into the office and sat down at the guest chair at my desk. "Close the door, Joseph," he said to me.

"Sure," I said as I closed the door and then walked to my desk. "What can I do for you?" I asked as I sat down.

Mr. Rackman put his leg over the armchair and stroked his genital area over his zipper. "I see you spend a lot of your time with the ladies here in the building. You have to be careful here. A lot of them come across as gay guys best friends but they're just gossips."

"Mr. Rackman," I said firmly, "you are making me very uncomfortable. Please put your leg down and stop rubbing on your genitals."

His face reddened and he stared at me with a deep angry stare. His eyebrows clenched hard. "Are you saying I'm coming on to you right now? You should know that one of the staff members here is accusing you of sexual harassment."

"Oh, which one? Is that why you are here?"

"No, that's not why I'm here. I wanted to check in with you. I hear you are doing a great job."

"I see. Well, what specifically would you like to know about the building?"

It never occurred to me to go back and ask him about the allegation he lodged my direction. "Look, the financial statements have to be signed this evening. I'm going around to make sure that everyone has had time to get to review them and get them signed."

"Mr. Rackman, I wasn't here during that timeframe. I will need over a month to go back and audit all of the documents to support that statement. Check with Shmuey and have him sign the statement to make it go faster."

"No! Shmuey isn't the administrator. You are. And, it is your job to sign them," he sternly said. I now knew why he was here at this building. This was the bullying session.

"I'll take a look at them tonight," I said without making any promises.

"Good," and he strolled out of the door. "Jane, your desk is a fucking mess. Do something about that," he said to her as he marched out of the door.

I walked over to Jane's desk and said, "Your desk looks fine. Don't worry about him. I'm not sure why he is in such a cranky mood."

"Dr. Wellington, he is always in a cranky mood."

Post Resignation

As some of you may be wondering, after my resignation I lodged more complaints against the facility. This was not out of anger, bitterness, or spite. I was legitimately concerned about the patients of the facility.

The facility was sold to another owner/operator within six months of my departure and many changes have been made.

I have been subpoenaed for many lawsuits that remain pending against the original nursing home owner. In one instance, the attorney representing the company asked me if I had any positive things to say about the company and I responded, "I don't think you are going to want me to be a part of this case. You see, I'm going to be honest about what happened at this building and the patterns that emerged that ultimately resulted in the litigation in the first place."

The attorney said he would call me back. He never did. Instead he emailed me with the following:

Dr. Wellington,

I met with my client and he has decided to settle out of court with the plaintiff.
Thank you for your help.

I often wondered how I was helpful. But, I realized something. I was able to help at least one person.

In another instance, I was asked to assist a family that had filed a lawsuit against the facility. Their mother had been brutally beaten to death by a resident that was 'schizophrenic' and had been refusing his medication. She was murdered in the facility and the records all indicated that the facility knew he was growing more violent. In my history, nursing homes don't discharge the residents to the hospital for psychiatric help to avoid losing daily payments on those residents.

Ultimately, I was able to work closely with a contact inside the facility still to obtain those records and send them via post to the family. The family ultimately won the lawsuit. They collected a tremendous amount of money but lost a loved one. There is no tradeoff for human life.

After many years of working as a nursing home administrator, I ultimately decided to consult for attorneys working on nursing home cases and have been very busy. Attorneys often hire 'legal nurse consultants' and the like but these people rarely know where to look to unlock the issues that caused situations. They look at the recorded data and draw conclusions. Attorneys I work with need to establish patterns to ensure nursing homes pay for the damage that they cause.

Make no mistake about it, nursing homes are essential to our future. But, my goal in life now is to make sure that I help get them on the 'straight and narrow'. I can only look forward now.

Now that you, the reader, are aware of serious situations (and these, again, are not isolated to one facility), you know where to look to help loved ones. You'll be helping the nursing home in the process, as well as all of the patients there.

I may be reached at JWellingtonPhD@gmail.com for future conversations and respond to emails as fast I am able to do so. Thank you for reading.